Culture and Curing

Culture and Curing

Anthropological Perspectives on
Traditional Medical Beliefs and Practices

EDITED BY

PETER MORLEY AND ROY WALLIS

UNIVERSITY OF PITTSBURGH PRESS

First published in Great Britain 1978 by Peter Owen Ltd
Published in the U.S.A. 1979 by the University of Pittsburgh Press
© Peter Morley and Roy Wallis 1978

Printed in Great Britain by
Daedalus Press Stoke Ferry King's Lynn Norfolk

Library of Congress Catalogue Card Number 78-62194
ISBN 0-8229-1136-1

Contents

Acknowledgments

Without exception, the papers in this volume are published here for the first time.

The editors would like to thank David Hughes and Vit Bubenik for their helpful comments on the manuscript. We are also indebted to Gwen McCauley, Cynthia Neary and Karen Tucker for their secretarial assistance in the preparation of this volume.

P.M. and R.W.

Peter Morley

1

Culture and the Cognitive World of Traditional Medical Beliefs: Some Preliminary Considerations

Let me begin by reminding you of the fact that the possession of true thoughts means everywhere the possession of invaluable instruments of action. . . .

William James,
Pragmatism, Lecture VI:
'Pragmatism's conception of truth'.

Ce qui est vrai à la lampe n'est pas toujours vrai au soleil.

Joubert, *Pensées, No. 152.*

One must seriously ask oneself whether superstition and myth, in the derogatory or non-scientific connotations of these words, are not due to our judging a given people from our conceptual standpoint, rather than theirs. . . . When the trouble was taken to find their concepts, then it became evident that everything made sense and that their behaviour and cultural norms followed as naturally and consistently from their particular categories of natural experience as ours do from our own. I believe it is just as much an error to suppose that there was no people anywhere who insisted on empirically, and hence scientifically, verified basic concepts before Galileo. Prevalent as the latter belief is, it is nonetheless rubbish.

F. S. C. Northrop.

1

The cognitive world of traditional societies tends to be less compartmentalized than that of the modern Western world. One aspect of life is usually inextricably intertwined with many others, not only situationally, but in the thought of those who inhabit technologically less developed societies. This book focuses on one aspect of life in non-Western societies, that of beliefs and practices relating to medical care. Historically, anthropologists have subsumed such beliefs or practices under some broader domain, such as religion, magic, or witchcraft. A simple typology of theories of disease causation readily shows why this should be so.

The diagnostic categories of disease causality reflect the extension of medicine into the broader social arena and the identification and classification of symptoms, social factors, and the perception of the practitioner.[1] These, while diverse in both form and content, may be subsumed under four broad categories (Figure 1).[2]

Supernatural causes	Non-Supernatural causes
Ultimate causes	Immediate causes

FIGURE 1: ETIOLOGICAL CATEGORIES

In the constructs represented in Figure 1, supernatural causes are those which place the origin of the disease with suprasensible forces, malevolent agents or acts which are not directly observable.[3] Within this category are found explanations such as *witchcraft* and *sorcery, spirit* or *demon intrusion, susto,* and *evil eye* to name but a few. Such explanations of disease causation are widely found in non-Western societies and have perhaps attracted most attention due to their radical divergence from those prevailing in modern Western medical science.

Non-supernatural disease etiologies are those based wholly on observed cause-and-effect relationships regardless of the accuracy of the observations made.[4] The diagnosis that an individual's malaise is due to profuse bleeding resulting from a wound is based on a non-supernatural theory of causation as is the observation that this same individual dies as a consequence of a swelling, located at the point of lesion, which moved up to his heart thereby killing him.[5]

The category of immediate causes follows from the non-supernatural explanations and accounts for disease and sickness in terms of perceived pathogenic agents. Ultimate causes explain the fundamentals which 'govern and condition the occurrence of disease'.[6] In short, immediate causes explain *how* diseases materialize, and ultimate causes *why* they happen.

Valabrega has suggested that there are essentially two conceptual frameworks found at work within traditional medical belief systems. These he refers to as the *endogenous* and *exogenous* concepts.[7] In the former (also termed centrifugal or subtractive) illness is caused by the magical capture of the individual's soul. The soul, which has left the individual's body, enters another realm, and the individual suffers as a result. Treatment involves magical intervention to recapture the soul, thereby restoring the balance of spiritual forces within the individual. In the case of the latter conception of disease, illness is caused by the intrusion of either a real or symbolic object into the patient's body. As such objects can range from thorns and small pebbles to rocks and small animals, we find here an example of a possible combination of supernatural and empirical causality. Only the specific object, in the presence or absence of some other factor, will determine which causal explanation achieves dominance. Thus, a small thorn producing an infection (natural) may be complemented by a supernatural explanation (the 'why?' dimension) where magical powers are attributed to either the offending object or some powerful force which moved the object towards its location in the individual's body. Here, as elsewhere, both *ultimate* and *immediate* causal explanations are offered and may lead to a combination of magical and empirical therapeutic endeavour.

In cases where spirits or demons enter the body, treatment follows from diagnostic pronouncements which suggest that supernatural forces have taken over and must be propitiated or exorcized through an appropriate ritual wherein the malevolent spirit is adjured to depart. Frequently, emetics are used to induce the vomiting away of the spirit. Also, we find a number of other physical treatments employed. These consist of 'sweating out' the

spirit, freezing, dietary measures and surgery – particularly tre-
panation.

Found throughout the vast range of traditional medical systems
are many beliefs and practices which contain an element of techno-
empirical knowledge.[8] For example, it has been suggested that the
acquisition of anatomical knowledge began very early in the
history of man and is closely related to the evolution of the car-
nivorous diet and its accompanying hunting activities.[9] Certainly,
for the Eskimo, long experience with the dressing of animals has
taught him a valuable lesson in gross and comparative anatomy.
Similarly, the development of so-called 'primitive technology',
much of which is biologically, as well as culturally adaptive, produced knowledge which was both biologically useful (in terms of
survival) and medically sophisticated.[10] For example, the development of clothing technology among polar and circumpolar peoples
must be seen as an important part of innovative human adaptation. Also, the use of medicinal plants to ward off scurvy, the avoidance of certain noxious food substances (e.g. polar bear liver), para-
site control, incest taboos, and other useful biologically adaptive
techniques may be seen as having an empirical component.[11]

Other widespread traditional medical practices include fasting,
blood letting, massage, isolation and confinement of pregnant
women, use of hot springs or mineral baths, steam baths, obstetrical
aid, detection of twins prior to birth, abortion and infanticide, and
special exercises to improve strength, dexterity and endurance.[12]
Medical practices requiring both anatomical knowledge and some
considerable degree of technical skill are trephining, caesarean
section, obstetrics, acupuncture, bonesetting, ligation, cauterization
and amputation, laparotomy, uvulectomy, removal of ovaries,
inoculation, inhalations, enemas, ointments and numerous herbal
treatments.[13] One finds an equally wide range of physical treatments, including electric shock therapy (the Abassines of Ethiopia
used electric catfish), sweat baths, and massage techniques, in the
area of traditional psychotherapy.[14]

The pharmacopoeia of traditional medicine is copious.[15] Among
the many drugs employed by traditional practitioners are quinine,
opium, coca, cinchona, copaiba, curare, chaulmoogra oil, ephe-
drine and rauwolfia.[16] In an impressive appendix, Vogel identifies
approximately 170 drugs which have been or remain officially in
the *National Formulary* or the *Pharmacopoeia of the United*

States of America which were used medicinally by North American Native Peoples north of Mexico; and about fifty more were used by inhabitants of the West Indies, Mexico, and Central and South America.[17]

There can be little doubt that traditional medicine has a complex *materia medica,* as both this brief overview and the papers presented in this volume attest. It is also certain that some measure of scientific status must be recognized in addition to the plethora of magico-religious beliefs and practices found throughout traditional cultures. Thus, while herbalist surgeons in Ethiopia mix mysticism (the name of the curative plant must not be said aloud) with the more pragmatic aspects of treatment, the *in toto* therapy does contain empirical qualities which have been experimentally tested over time.[18]

To further our understanding of traditional medical beliefs and practices, it is essential to grasp their phenomenological and social meanings. These meanings are rendered intelligible 'in terms of the expectations of the actors, the narrative-building character of disease etiologies, and the processual nature of cures'.[19] Moreover, this means that analysis must focus on what people hope for and expect from their medical system, as well as what they define as etiologically significant and as therapeutically efficacious.[20]

The papers included in this volume are directed towards exploring some of these intelligible connections and their social meaning. We wish to prepare these substantive analyses with some consideration of the dominant conceptualizations of non-Western medical practice which have prevailed in the accounts of medical historians and anthropologists. Since much of this attention has been directed specifically at supernaturalistic explanations of illness, particularly in terms of witchcraft, it is upon these that we shall focus.

Western allopathic medicine, as a social institution, has, over the past half a century, achieved a dominant position in the provision of health care. The corpus of empirical knowledge, recognized as the *materia medica* of the Western physician, and developed particularly in the context of the scientific revolution, has emerged as the *sine qua non* of 'legitimate' medical practice.

Throughout the history of Western medicine, with a few exceptions, there has been a tendency to view traditional medical systems and beliefs from the vantage point of contemporary Western medical science, regarding them as not only 'primitive', but archaic and largely irrelevant to both scientific medicine and the health of human populations. The emphasis has been on the quaint, but queer, customs and lore of the 'savage'. Imbued with the idea of progress, physicians, medical historians, and early anthropologists viewed 'primitive' medicine as an early stage in evolutionary development. Traditional medicine, even as currently practised in many non-Western societies, was therefore seen as a simple predecessor of complex modern scientific medicine.[28]

The success of positivistically-based science as measured popularly by technological achievement has resulted in the Western scientific world view achieving a paramount position as the uniquely legitimate interpreter of nature.

> Whereas alternatives to our presently-constructed social order are usually found threatening and dangerous, such is the confidence engendered by our conceptions of natural order that alternatives to them are merely treated as odd, or perhaps amusing. And no powerful social group or society exists with an alternative natural world view that may serve to shake our faith in our own. Quaint cosmologies in our midst, or the anthropomorphic physics of primitive societies, disturb us no more often than the existence of those who believe in them. Whereas we like to think our values are the best, we know our view of nature is the right one.[22]

That phenomena which do not fit prevailing scientific paradigms are often rejected as 'unscientific', 'pre-scientific', or 'pre-logical' is well documented. Of particular importance here is the work of Lévy-Bruhl, whose reflections on the pre-logical and mystical nature of primitive belief systems exercised considerable influence on early (and to some extent even on later) anthropological explanations of *'la pensée sauvage'*.

Lévy-Bruhl insisted that there were fundamental differences between the pre-logical, animistic, and anti-experimental mentality of primitive man and 'those characteristic of "scientific thinking"'.[23] He contrasted the 'mystical *aspect* of primitive mentality' with the rational aspect of 'scientific society'.[24] The fuller ramifications of his thesis suggest that:

> . . . the reality in which primitives move is itself mystical. There is not a being, not an object, not a natural phenomenon that

appears in their collective representations in the way that it appears to us. Almost all that we see therein escapes them, or is a matter of indifference to them. On the other hand, they see many things of which we are unaware.[25]

Essentially, he argues, the thought of primitive man is pre-logical. That is to say:

it is not constrained above all else, as ours is, to avoid contradictions. The same logical exigencies are not in its case always present. What to our eyes is impossible or absurd, it sometimes will admit without seeing any difficulty.[26]

It is somewhat unfortunate that Lévy-Bruhl chose the term 'pre-logical' to describe primitive mentality, for he clearly did not mean to imply that primitive thought was illogical, but rather that it was not in accord with the 'rationalist' logic of Western thought. Moreover, primitive thought obeys a 'law of participation'. Hence:

. . . In the collective representations of primitive mentality, objects, beings, phenomena, can, in a fashion incomprehensible to us, be at the same time themselves and something other than themselves.[27]

Moreover, they can be joined by connections which have nothing in common with the logic of the Western tradition of philosophical and scientific rationalism.[28] The pre-logical thought of the primitive is indifferent to such logic and dispenses with the principles of contradictions and causality. In sum, 'logically' separate aspects of reality merge into a single mystic unity. It is thus not difficult to derive from Lévy-Bruhl's account the notion that primitive thought is essentially inferior to Western thought.

Taking issue with Lévy-Bruhl, Evans-Pritchard has argued against the notion of pre-logical mentality. Commenting specifically on this theory, he asserts that the scientific world view is as much a function of culture as is the magical perspective of the 'savage', a function of 'primitive' culture.[29] Evans-Pritchard clarifies his position as follows:

The fact that we attribute rain to meteorological causes alone, while savages believe that Gods, or ghosts, or magic can in-

fluence the rainfall, is no evidence that our brains function
differently from their brains. It does not show that we 'think
more logically' than savages, at least not if this expression suggests some kind of hereditary psychic superiority. It is no sign of
superior intelligence on my part that I attribute rain to physical
causes. I did not come to this conclusion myself by observation
and inference and have, in fact, little knowledge of the meteorological process that leads to rain. I merely accept what every-
body else in my society accepts, namely that rain is due to
natural causes. This particular idea formed part of my culture
long before I was born into it and little more was required of me
than sufficient linguistic ability to learn it. Likewise, a savage,
who believes that under suitable natural and ritual conditions
the rainfall can be influenced by use of appropriate magic, is
not on account of this belief to be considered of inferior intelligence. He did not build up this belief from his own observations
and inferences but adopted it in the same way as he adopted the
rest of his cultural heritage, namely by being born into it. He
and I are both thinking in patterns of thought provided for us by
the societies in which we live.

It would be absurd to say that the savage is thinking mysti-
cally and that we are thinking scientifically about rainfall. In
either case, like mental processes are involved; and, moreover,
the content of thought is similarly derived. But, we can say that
the social content of our thought about rainfall is scientific, is in
accord with objective facts, whereas the social content of savage
thought about rainfall is unscientific, since it is not in accord
with reality and may also be mystical where it assumes the
existence of supra-sensible forces.[30]

Evans-Pritchard has distinguished here between thought-as-
process and the social content of thought. Explanations of the
natural order of things, as presented by primitive thought systems,
while often false, are, Evans-Pritchard concedes, based on observation; but, while taxonomies of phenomena are developed by loca-
ting their similarities (as in empirical science), the 'magician' differs
from the scientist in inferring that because things are alike in one or
more respects, they have a mystical link between them whereas, in
fact, the link is not a real link but an ideal connection in the mind
of the magician.[31]

The example of African witchcraft, the essence of Evans-
Pritchard's contribution to current philosophical debate on the

problem of rationality, serves to illustrate the extent of observation and logic inherent in traditional medical belief systems.

As Evans-Pritchard and others have shown, witchcraft may be seen as a cultural knowledge system with its own internal coherence and plausibility.[32] In this sense, it has been argued that witchcraft is 'quite similar to the cultural knowledge systems of modern science in terms of certain general structural features. . .'.[33] They are similar 'in that they possess "elegant" internal organizational patterns, and in their superbly effective adaptation to whatever factual realities may be recognized in the given context'.[34] Clearly, there are differences between these two cosmologies; but, in both cases, they are firmly rooted in socio-cultural contexts.[35]

A system of scientific ideas combines two essential characteristics, 'abstractness' and 'testability'. The former is related to the internal organization of the system of ideas, while the latter 'pertains to the system's relation to external facts'.[36] Moreover:

> *Abstractness* means that the logical aspects of the system's internal organization are differentiated from the factual content of the system: that logical relationships among the component propositions are clarified and that the most general propositions of the system pertain to principles or laws to be applied under hypothetical circumstances, rather than to concrete factual situations. *Testability* means that the system provides a basis for predicting observable outcomes, and hence, that it is subject to evaluation in terms of the accuracy of its predictions.[37]

Richter goes on to warn us that:

> Either abstractness or testability may be present without the other. . . . In fact, abstractness and testability are relatively difficult to combine because abstractness means that a system, if it is to be testable, can be tested only under special conditions which must usually be artificially constructed. Specifically, the combination of abstractness and testability, which marks a system as 'scientific', means that the system predicts certain observable outcomes, rather than others not under ordinary or natural conditions, but under ideal conditions of observational or experimental control. . . .[38]

Such a broad definition of a scientific system does not focus on the *content* of the system itself – its ideational characteristics. Rather, the emphasis is on the *structural* features as *the markers* of a scientific thought system.

Richter offers a series of propositions which illustrate the 'scientific' status of witchcraft belief systems and the etiology of sickness. His hypothetical people believe that:

a) witchcraft produces illness in people;
b) illness is produced *only* by witchcraft;
c) magical defences against witchcraft protect potential victims from witch-induced illness;
d) illness can be warded off *only* by magical intervention.[39]

This abstract belief system, Richter concludes, informs us of what will happen under 'certain conditions of perfect experimental control: victims of witchcraft who are not protected by magic will fall ill.'[40] Also, the system is clearly testable in principle: 'we could attempt to make someone ill via witchcraft, prevent the use of defensive magic, and see if he falls ill, as the system would predict under these conditions.'[41]

How, then, does a witchcraft system, located in the real world, differ from the above hypothetical construct? In what ways is a witchcraft belief system not 'scientific'? First, everyday witchcraft systems are usually stated in terms of *in situ* events. That is to say, when visible and not worked in secret, we can see that X invoked witchcraft to produce illness in Y. The causal factor is describable at a non-abstract level of meaning. However, the proposition 'if X then Y' is rarely formulated:[42]

'If witchcraft and no defensive magic, then illness – are ordinarly not formulated by believers in such a system, even though the external observer from a scientificially advanced culture may recognize such ideas as implicitly underlying the concrete statements and the behaviour of the believers.[43]

We also find a second distinguishing characteristic. The witchcraft belief system is also unlikely to be testable in the 'real' world of the believer. Once again, the problem appears to be related to the existence of unclear criteria for determining whether or not witchcraft was in fact the 'cause' of an individual's illness.[44] As

with other belief systems, the efficacy of a witchcraft system is difficult to challenge or refute. Indeed, its failure may be attributed to
the existence of powerful, defensive magic carried out in secret, or
the errors made in the practical aspect of witchcraft ritual and
process.[45] Furthermore, witchcraft explanations are rarely, if ever,
seen as *in toto* explanations of misfortune. Indeed, frequently they
are seen as necessary, but not sufficient, causal explanations of
events. In every case of misfortune and malaise, there is a 'how?'
and a 'why?' to be answered.[46] And, as Gluckman observes, the
African 'distinguishes the why and the how of misfortunes as
clearly as we do'.[47] This point will be taken up again later in this
chapter.

Believers in witchcraft causality are not satisfied with explanations which do not go beyond informing them *how* a certain misfortune or illness occurred. Thus, when a farmer blames a witch for
the failure of his crops, or a hunter is killed by an elephant, or when
men sit on a termite-infested granary and are killed by the structure's collapse, there is then a search for meaning. This search takes
the believers in the direction of the witchcraft system which
answers the question 'why?' Also asked are the questions: 'Why
this granary?', 'Why this hunter?', 'Why at this particular time?'
And, as Gluckman comments:

> Witchcraft is, thus, a theory of causation; but, it is a theory
> which explains causal links which modern scientists do not
> attempt, cannot attempt, to explain. Other people ascribe the
> particularity of phenomena to ancestor spirits, providence, Kis-
> met, the will or retribution of God; the skeptical scientist can
> only say it is chance, the coincidence of two chains of events in
> space-time.[48]

Again:

> The belief in witchcraft thus provides explanations for the par-
> ticularity of misfortunes. It does not, for the African, provide
> the whole interpretation of the misfortune. The belief in witch-
> craft does not exclude empirical observation and scientific
> understanding; on the contrary, witchcraft belief embraces and
> uses empirical observation and scientific understanding. The
> witch has to cause misfortune through disease, termites eating
> wood, elephants, crop blight; and all these exist in their own

right and have their own effects on men's lives.[49]

The Azande, then, see no contradictions in their notions of causality. There is always an explanation ready to account for a contradiction or any predictive failure of the oracle. Evans-Pritchard refers to the 'secondary elaboration of belief'[50] where Azande explain the failure of the oracle in as many as eight different ways. These explanations consist, among others, of assumptions that the wrong poison was used, a breach of taboo committed, or that the poison was spoiled, and so on. Azande, states Evans-Pritchard, are firm in their beliefs:

> They reason excellently in the idiom of their beliefs, but they cannot reason outside, or against, their beliefs because they have no other idiom in which to express their thoughts.[51]

This extreme position has been more recently emphasized by Robin Horton, who places the traditional thinker completely and inextricably within the idiom of his culture:

> In traditional cultures, there is no developed awareness of alternatives to the established body of theoretical tenets. . . .[52]

Contrary, then, to scientifically orientated cultures, traditional thought systems are seen by Horton to offer no alternative theoretical tenets to explain away phenomena:

> In these traditional cultures, questioning of the beliefs on which divining is based and weighing up of success against failures are just not among the paths that thought can take. They are blocked paths because the thinkers involved are victims of the closed predicament. For them, established beliefs have an absolute validity, and any threat to such beliefs is a horrific threat of chaos.[53]

Doubtless, some individuals do hold 'uncritical' attitudes to conceptual systems. Such conceptual loyalty does exist. But, reasons Gellner, 'consider the implications of accepting this as a general criterion of traditional mentality':

> . . . It means that within it, there can be no syncretism, no doc-

trinal pluralism, no deep treason, no dramatic conversion or doctrinal oscillation, no holding of alternative belief-systems up one's sleeve, ready for the opportune moment of betrayal.[54]

Horton's position is absolutist and ultimately a philosophy of individualism.[55] The 'awareness of alternatives' appears to be credited to individuals alone.[56] Thus, Horton's psychologistic reasoning permits only the individual deviant the option of alternative realities. His position, and an influential one at that, is that traditional thought systems are, in Popper's terms, 'closed' and permit no alternative explanations other than those derived from the established body of theoretical tenets which form the cultural *eidos* of a given people. However, there are clearly many cultures where a plurality of belief systems in general and of medical beliefs in particular are found. As Daryll Forde says:

> It is not to be assumed that the views and attitudes of a people concerning the duties of men among themselves and their relations to the universe are necessarily all of one piece. Anthropological studies of many cultures have shown that even in small and comparatively isolated societies where differences of wealth, rank, and power are small, there need be no complete integration of belief and doctrine, still less the domination of conduct in all spheres by a single system of beliefs or basic ideas. For both the historical sources of knowledge and belief and the contexts of activity in which these are evoked are likely, even in a circumscribed world, to be diverse. On the other hand, there is reason to believe that a close relation exists between dominant attitudes towards social relations and the proper use of resources and established beliefs concerning the nature of human society and its place in a wider universe of cosmic forces. Between such beliefs and their opportunities for action, there appears to be a continuous process of reciprocal adjustment.[57]

Thus, while Horton's observation that belief systems are culture-bound and are to be examined for logic and rationality within this context, requires serious consideration, considerable evidence suggests that his notion of the 'optionless' world of the traditional thinker with its closed thought system must be questioned.

Horton's major contribution to our understanding of traditional belief systems is his elaboration of Popper's 'situational logic' as it applies to human thought and its conceptual development. In the case of medical belief systems, he suggests that the validity of Western or African theories of illness is *always* relative to the conditions in which these occur. He postulates that traditional *theories* of disease causation take the thinker beyond the level of commonsense reasoning and produce a far wider cosmology of disease categories.

The traditional thinker and the Western scientist both use theory 'to transcend the limited vision of natural causes provided by commonsense'. Thus, states Horton, when a diviner diagnoses the action of witchcraft influence as the causal factor in a client's illness, it is a central part of his *modus operandi* to add something about jealousies, misdeeds, or malevolent human relations. Similarly, should the diviner indicate that his client has incurred the wrath of his ancestors, he will add the observation that there has been a breach of kinship morality and it is this offence which has precipitated the client's malaise. The parallel between the diviner and the scientist, at the level of situational logic, is further elaborated by Horton:

> The situation is not very different from that in which a puzzled American layman, seeing a large mushroom cloud on the horizon, consults a friend who happens to be a physicist. On the one hand, the physicist may refer him to theoretical entities. 'Why this cloud? Well, a massive fusion of hydrogen nuclei has just taken place.' Pushed further, however, the physicist is likely to refer to the assemblage and dropping of a bomb containing special substances. Substitute 'disease' for 'mushroom cloud', 'spirit anger' for 'massive fusion of hydrogen nuclei', *and we are back again with the diviner.* In both cases, reference to theoretical entities is used to link events to the visible, tangible world (natural effects) to their antecedents in the same world (natural causes).[58]

Within the context of the witchcraft belief system, the emphasis is on disturbed personal relations. And, as Horton remarks, modern Western medicine, blinded by the success of the germ theory of disease, has for a long time ignored the relationship between social disturbance and individual affliction. Of course, contemporary allopathy is now more fully aware of the nexus between social disturbance and illness, and this growing interest is reflected in the development of psychosomatic medicine. Certainly, when juxta-posed to the notions of psychosomatic medicine and other dimensions of post-Cartesian thought, the ancestor-spirit/witchcraft theory of illness causation, emphasizing the quality of the patient's social relations, does not appear as fatuous as at first glance. Even at the level of disease caused by infecting micro-organisms, 'bad social relations could well tip the scales one way or the other'.[59]

When we examine a patient from the vantage point of Western allopathic medicine, for example, we 'know' that he is sick, because our sophisticated laboratory techniques show that he is infected by *Clostridium tetani* and that his malaise is the result of a deep puncture wound which permitted anaerobic bacteria to enter his bloodstream. For those who embrace supernatural theories of causation, this process goes unnoticed. Within the context of the supernatural, witchcraft, 'evil eye', or 'bad air' may be isolated as the offending agents; whereas, for those who accept non-supernatural theories of causality, the blame is placed on invading bacteria, viruses, germs, etc. In this latter category, modern industrial man generally turns to empirical theories of disease etiology, although this is certainly not the only path to diagnosis and treatment found in such societies. Moreover, while industrial man may well be informed as to the existence of such pathogenic factors as bacteria, germs, and viruses, it is doubtful if many individuals are that well informed that they fully comprehend the structure, function, and general physiological effects of such pathogenic organisms. Rarely has the esoterica of Western medicine and science percolated down to the commonsense level of reality without a concomitant dilution of factual content and the incorporation of some degree of mysticism and 'magic'. Thus, while modern industrial man submits to the scientifically-based *materia medica* of the allopathic physician, it does not necessarily follow that the former understands either the knowledge behind medical practice and its nosology, or the complexity of treatments offered him by the latter. In essence, the allopath's patient, is, like the Zande, a participant in a belief system. Perhaps the essential difference is that the Azande are more involved in, and less mystified by, both the belief system itself and the diagnostic utterances of its practitioners than are the patients within the Western allopathic medical context.

'Medicine', in the ethnomedical sense, is to be seen as more than the fiat of the Western medical paradigm.[60] The really fundamental *sine qua non* of medicine in both traditional and modern industrial societies is that it is a social phenomenon and can only be fully understood as such. In traditional societies medical knowledge is far more closely integrated with the institutions and all-encompassing cosmology of the society as a whole than is the case in more differentiated industrial societies.[61] It is this feature of traditional medical systems, holding in obeyance the issue of 'truth' and 'efficacy', which the essays in this volume seek to explore.

NOTES AND REFERENCES

1   A. Alland, Jr., *Adaptation in Cultural Evolution: An Approach to Medical Anthropology,* New York, Columbia University Press, 1970, p. 138.

2   The categories in Figure 1 are derived from those of Evans-Pritchard and Seijas.

3   H. Seijas, 'An approach to the study of the medical aspects of culture', *Current Anthropology,* December 1973, pp. 544-5.

4   Ibid.

5   Ibid.

6   Ibid.

7   J. P. Valabrega, *La Relation Thérapeutique: Malade et Médecin,* Paris, Flammarion, 1962.

8   W. Laughlin, 'Primitive theory of medicine: empirical knowledge', in I. Galdston (ed.), *Man's Image in Medicine and Anthropology,* New York, International Universities Press, 1963, p. 116.

9   Ibid., p. 118.

10   Ibid., p. 119.

11   Ibid.

12   Ibid.

13   Ibid. See also E. H. Ackerknecht, *Medicine and Ethnology, Selected Essays,* Baltimore, The Johns Hopkins University Press, 1971.

14   The reader who wishes to read further on the subject of traditional psychiatric diagnosis and treatment is referred to J. Kennedy, 'Cultural psychiatry', in J. Honigmann (ed.), *Handbook of Social and Cultural Anthropology,* Chicago, Rand McNally College Publishing Company, 1974, pp. 1119-98; A. Kiev, *Magic, Faith and Healing,* New York, The Free Press, 1964; E. Fuller Torrey, *The Mind Game,* New York, Bantam Books, 1972.

15   R. Lieban, 'Medical anthropology', in Honigmann, op. cit., pp. 1031-72. This chapter is an excellent overview of the field.

16   Ibid., p. 1045.

17   V. Vogel, *American Indian Medicine,* New York, Ballantine Books, 1970 (see especially pp. 253-401).

18   Lieban, op. cit., p. 1045.

19   A. Young, 'Some implications of medical beliefs and practices for Social Anthropology', *American Anthropologist,* Vol. 78, No. 1, March 1976, pp. 5-24.

20   Ibid., p. 20.

21   See E. H. Ackerknecht, op. cit.; H. Sigerist, *Primitive and Archaic Medicine,* New York, Oxford University Press, 1967.

22   B. Barnes, *Scientific Knowledge and Sociological Theory,* London, Routledge & Kegan Paul, 1974, p. 2.

23   S. Lukes, 'Some problems about rationality', in B. Wilson (ed.), *Rationality,* Oxford, Basil Blackwell, 1970, p. 201.

24   Ibid.

25   L. Lévy-Bruhl, *Les Fonctions Mentales dans les Sociéties Inférieures,* Paris, 1910, p. 20 (cited in S. Lukes, op. cit., p. 201).

26   Idem, *La Mentalité Primitive,* Oxford, 1931, p. 21 (in Lukes, op. cit., p. 201).

27   Idem, in J. Cazeneuve, *Lucien Lévy-Bruhl: Sa Vie, Son Oeuvre avec un Exposé de sa Philosophie,* Paris, Collections Philosophes, 1965, p. 80. See also the review article by D. Goddard, *Social Research,* June 1967, pp. 384-7.

28   D. Goddard, op. cit., p. 385.

29   Cf. P. Winch, 'Understanding a primitive society', in B. Wilson, op. cit., p. 79; M. Richter, *Science as a Cultural Process,* London, Frederick Muller, 1973, especially pp. 43-52; B. Barnes, op. cit., passim.

30   E. Evans-Pritchard, 'Lévy-Bruhl's theory of primitive mentality', *Bulletin of the Faculty of Arts,* University of Egypt, 1934 (in Winch, op. cit., pp. 79-80).

31   Idem, in Lukes, op. cit., pp. 198-9.

32   See M. Richter, op. cit., pp. 43-52. Cultural knowledge systems, as defined by Richter, refer to 'any set of ideas, prevailing in a given culture or subculture, which provides a way of organizing information about the world or about any aspect of it' (p. 43).

33   Ibid., p. 46.

34   Ibid.

35   We refer here to the 'social construction of reality' thesis advanced by P. Berger and T. Luckmann in *The Social Construction of Reality: A Treatise in the Sociology of Knowledge,* New York, Doubleday, 1966.

36   Richter, op. cit., p. 47.

37 Ibid.

38 Ibid., pp. 47-8.

39 Ibid., p. 48.

40 Ibid.

41 Ibid., p. 46.

42 Ibid.

43 Ibid.

44 Ibid.

45 Ibid.

46 M. Gluckman, 'Social beliefs and individual thinking in tribal society', in R. Manners and D. Kaplan (eds.), *Theory in Anthropology: A Sourcebook,* Chicago, Aldine Publishing Company, 1968, p. 455.

47 Ibid.

48 Ibid., p. 456.

49 Ibid. (emphasis added).

50 E. Evans-Pritchard, *Witchcraft, Oracles and Magic Among the Azande,* Oxford, Clarendon Press, 1937, p. 330.

51 Ibid., p. 338.

52 R. Horton, 'African traditional thought and western science', in B. Wilson, loc. cit., pp. 131-71.

53 Ibid., p. 163.

54 E. Gellner, *Legitimation of Belief,* London, Cambridge University Press, 1974, p. 156.

55 Ibid., p. 157.

56 Ibid.

57 D. Forde (ed.), *African Worlds: Studies in the Cosmological and Social Values of African Peoples,* London, Oxford University Press, 1968, p. vii.

58 Horton, op. cit., p. 136 (emphasis added).

59 M. G. Marwick, 'Witchcraft and the epistemology of science', Presidential Address to Section N of the British Association for the Advancement of Science, Stirling, Scotland, 1974, p. 10.

60 Young, op. cit., p. 6.

61 Ibid. See also H. Fabrega, 'Some features of Zincantecan medical knowledge', *Ethnology,* Vol. 10, 1971, pp. 25-43; idem, 'The study of medical problems in preliterate settings', *Yale Journal of Biology and Medicine,* Vol. 43, 1971, pp. 385-407.

Michael Kearney

2

Spiritualist Healing in Mexico[1]

In the mid 1800s, an ecstatic movement known variously as spiritualism or spiritism spread throughout much of Europe and the
Americas. Although dressed in modern garb, spiritualism-spiritism
represents an archaic stratum of human religious thought and
action, the essential features of which are various altered states of
consciousness attributed to special human powers or contact with
spirit-beings. Belief in soul voyaging and spirit-familiars are other
typical traits. In Mexico these two mainstreams were strongly
affected by the folk culture and social milieu into which they were
introduced, subsequently developing into what is today a loosely
organized ecstatic religion focusing largely on folk healing, and
referred to generally as *espiritualismo* or *espiritismo*.[2] This paper is
based on an investigation of spiritualism done intermittently by the
author from 1968 to the present in and around the town of Ensenada, a port on the Pacific coast of northern Baja California, the
northwestern-most state of Mexico.

No attempt is made in the short confines of this paper to assess
precisely the effectiveness of spiritualist healing; rather I shall outline the relationships between folk medical concepts, symptoms,
and therapeutic responses. It should be noted, however, that signi-
cant alleviation of symptoms is obtained and that seeking such
relief is a major motivation for participation in *espiritualismo*.

Background Ethnography[3]

Ensenada is part of the western border region of northern Mexico which also includes the cities of Tijuana, Tecate and Mexicali. This area is currently one of the fastest growing urban regions in the world, with population increases of over 100 per cent every ten years typical of these cities. The state as a whole grew from 48,327 in 1930 to 870,421 in 1970, due largely to an influx of immigrants from mainland Mexico, seeking better economic conditions. In this area, spiritualism thrives in mushrooming neighbourhoods consisting mostly of jerry-built houses erected by squatters and other low-income residents new to the area. These communities of this 'frontier culture'[4] contrast with more stable Mexican towns and villages where social relationships are more extensive, and cultural traditions more homogenous and conservative.

✗ The most reasonable explanation for the presence of spiritualism among this population is that it is an adaptation to the relatively structureless and anomic conditions resulting from this rapid urbanization to which it responds by providing easily formed, flexible social networks in an urban society otherwise virtually lacking in social groupings other than the family.[5] It also, as I shall show below, responds to psychiatric symptoms of stress and alienation.

The focal points of spiritualist activities are called *templos* or *recintos,* of which I have made observations in ten of the dozen or so that are present in and around Ensenada. These 'temples' are typically small buildings especially constructed for this purpose with the appearance of a simple chapel. Each temple is founded by a spirit medium, known as a *materia,* who has done so at the command of a spirit-being which appeared to her during the course of an illness. Becoming a spirit medium and founding a temple are usually described as the fulfilment of an obligation incurred when healed.

A significant event in identifying oneself as a spiritualist is the acquisition of a spirit familiar with guardian or tutelary functions. But the main requirement for becoming a medium is the ability to 'open' one's body so that spirit-beings may enter into it and express themselves through it, almost invariably by using the medium's vocal organs. Bourguignon[6] refers to such behaviour and altered states of consciousness as 'possession trance', which she distinguishes from 'trance'. In *espiritualismo,* trance states include *videncia,* the ability to 'see' spirit phenomena with the eyes shut and at a distance; *clarividencia,* the ability to 'see' spirit phenomena with opened eyes; and *oido,* the ability to 'hear' spirit-beings. Some mediums and other 'less well developed' spiritualists who specialize in healing make use of a sort of X-ray *clarividencia* for diagnosis, that is, looking into someone 'to see the sickness' within them. Whereas possession trance involves an active performance, trance is typically a more passive experience.

As spiritualists conceptualize the world, it is charged with two major types of personal and impersonal forces. One type is the magical power of witches, who are believed to be commonly present in local neighbourhoods. The other, peculiar to spiritualism, consists of various spirit-beings who descend to this 'worldly plane' from some vaguely conceived ethereal realm. Of these there are two subtypes. First, in terms of reverence accorded them, are the Divinities (*Divinidades*), also known as The Four Powers (*Las Quatro Potencias*), which consist of Father God (*Padre Dios*), Father Jesus (*Padre Jesús*), Father Elijah (*Padre Elías,* also referred to as The White Dove, namely The Holy Spirit), and the Holy Mother (*La Madre Santísima*). These are not personalities so much as 'forces' or 'powers' which send their 'radiations' to 'penetrate' into the brains of mediums who then serve as their 'loudspeakers'. When they appear through revered mediums, the speech of the Divinities is typically rhythmic, sonorous and assertive, yet compassionate and tender. The male Divinities appear as very masculine and strong, whereas the Holy Mother, who appears only occasionally, has a less commanding presence.

The second subtype consists of 'spirits' or 'beings' *per se.* This is a heterogeneous assortment of good and bad spirits of, for the most part, deceased humans, including Christian saints, figures out of history, relatives of living spiritualists, foreigners, etc.; visitors from outer space, dwarfs, and so forth also appear. There are numerous such spirits which enter into mediums primarily to heal. Most often these healing spirits are the spirits of dead doctors, Indians, or Orientals.

For the truly visionary adepts this image of reality as charged with helpful versus harmful forces is confirmed by their *videncias* and *clarividencias*; for the nonvisionary, 'undeveloped' new initiates and peripheral participants, the recounted visionary experiences of others support this conception of the world.

Almost all temples have regularly scheduled activities at least several days a week. Of these the most important to spiritualists are *cátedras* (classes) and *curaciones* (healings). *Cátedras* are held on the 1st, 7th, 13th, and 21st of each month, and every Sunday morning. At these sessions any mediums present are possessed by the most prominent spirit-beings in the spiritualist pantheon. Speaking through the mediums these spirit-beings usually deliver what amounts to sermons. These 'doctrines' tend to be garbled and rambling, dwelling mainly on moral themes and exhorting the audience to persevere in their spiritual development. Healings are formally scheduled for Tuesdays and Fridays, but in practice the distinction between *cátedras* and *curaciones* is blurred in that healing is also often done at *cátedras* as well as at *curaciones*. At these meetings mediums, especially ones who work with familiars which specialize in healing, are possessed by these spirits which then treat the infirm and mentally disturbed. Other 'less developed' healers, who are capable of trance experiences, but who 'do not yet' enter into possession trance also heal at these sessions with the aid of healing spirits.

From biographies of adepts it is apparent that social status and illness are two major predisposing conditions in recruitment. First, within the general population described above, it is predominantly women who are attracted to spiritualism. One indicator of this sex imbalance is an overwhelmingly greater number of women attending spiritualist services. Also, of seventeen mediums known to me, sixteen are women. And as indicated above, these women are mostly from the lower classes. The second prevalent feature of initiates is sickness at the time of recruitment. Of thirty-six followers for whom I have biographical data, thirty-three became involved in spiritualism during an illness.

Sickness is pivotal in recruitment in that significant, often sudden symptom alleviation is a powerful reinforcement. The crisis state of illness with attendant anxiety exacerbated by financial and personal insecurities predisposes novices to a major cognitive restructuring in which former world-view assumptions and sense of self are altered to accord with the spiritualist cosmology.

Spiritualists tend to concentrate around particular mediums in core groups of fifteen to twenty, but membership is informal and loosely bounded. Most followers attach themselves primarily to one particular medium and her temple, but also visit others where they tend to be well received. Aside from the healing aspects of these voluntary associations, they provide mutual aid. When members need shelter or nursing care, they can turn to acquaintances within the spiritualist network, and, by virtue of this self-proclaimed membership, they can seek out other spiritualists when travelling or moving to other locales.

Spiritualist Healing

As is typical throughout the world where traditional healing systems exist alongside modern medical facilities, spiritualists tend to resort to the latter for major bodily traumas and severe infectious diseases, while seeking alleviation of ethnospecific syndromes and other symptoms primarily in the former. Occasionally people will avail themselves of both systems – simultaneously or sequentially – for a particular ailment.

These therapeutic strategies are based in part on empirical knowledge of the relative effectiveness of these alternatives for treatment of these two major categories of illnesses. Relative costs and access are also considerations in that spiritualist treatments are usually less expensive and more readily available than modern medical services. Finally, decisions to seek spiritual healing are influenced by assumptions about the causes of illness and their appropriate treatments; these etiological concepts are in turn consistent with basic assumptions in the spiritualist world view.

For cases in which they intervene, spiritualist healers invariably pronounce that the cause of the ailment is due to the intrusion into the invalid of some alien spirit or force. The first step in treatment is therefore indentification of this malignant influence. This diagnosis confirms the magical nature of the illness which the invalid already suspects, and thus from the point of view of scientific medicine could be seen as counterproductive. But as in perhaps all medical traditions, naming the causal agent reduces ambiguity and anxiety, and is thus the first step in curing. Also, from the invalid's point of view, this immediate diagnosis and ensuing treatment are superior to the often delayed pronouncement of a medical doctor who may have to wait for laboratory test results or consultations.

According to spiritualists, the single most important factor in healing is belief in the effectiveness of the cure. As one medium expressed this point, 'Nothing will be effective without faith [*fe*], not even the best doctors; but with sufficient faith one can be cured with plain water.' This insistence on the primacy of belief is common to both spiritualism and traditional Mexican folk medicine. Typically it is said that it is not faith in the curer or treatment *per se* which is necessary, but in God, who is responsible for their healing powers. Healing mediums assert that they cure 'in the name of God', and only if the client has sufficient faith in Him. One implication of this is that it allows placing the burden for failed cures on the client by arguing that he lacked sufficient faith.

Since belief in the reality of God, and in spiritualist principles and phenomena in general, is seen as necessary, it follows that doubt is believed to reduce the possibility of being healed. Spiritualists therefore attempt to dispel doubt and disbelief, both individually and collectively. The expectation of being cured certainly facilitates the cure of conversion reactions (see below). There are also two types of indirect evidence that belief figures in the course of both psychosomatic and more strictly organic conditions. One is the literature on belief in helplessness as a cause of psychogenic death due to cognitive arousal of the autonomic nervous system.[7] The other, which can be seen as the positive side of this coin, is the healing response due to the now well demonstrated placebo effect.[8]

Most Common Psychiatric Symptoms

BODILY COMPLAINTS

The vast majority of symptoms for which adepts seek spiritualist relief are a diverse assortment of aches, pains, and physical disabilities. Without clinical assessment it is impossible to determine the frequency of those which are due to organic versus psychological causes. It is certain, however, that the social conditions of *espiritualismo,* as described above, are conducive to a high incidence of the conversion reactions. Within the folk-medical knowledge there is little or no awareness of the mechanism of conversion, although folk etiology does rightly attribute many physical symptoms to strong emotional experiences. But instead of seeing such symptoms as due to stress which is symbolically and psychologically mediated, they are thought of as secondary symptoms due to some condition such as humoral imbalance (see below) which is caused by a primary natural or supernatural etiology. Spiritualist healing is, however, eminently suited for dealing with such symptoms, especially the conversion reactions. Its power resides in the complex of assumptions about illnesses, their causes and cures, and the ability of the healers to bring these assumptions to life as intensely experienced imagery, which for the most part is taken as real. The prime example of this is the performance of 'spiritual surgery', i.e. 'operations' conducted by 'spiritual doctors' working through mediums. These doctors are most often exotic spirits, usually of foreign nationality, and some of them are specialists in such things as ailments of the head (eye, ear, and nose), internal disorders, 'cancer', etc. They operate by entering into a medium with whom they have established a working relationship. The medium is in possession trance while the spirit is operating and, aside from mouthing verbal instructions given by the spirit, she does not act. In other words, it is the spirit himself who actually performs the operation, i.e. it is done invisibly, except to those who are able 'to see'. Often the 'patient' is granted this power so that he may observe the operation. If the patient does not actually see the procedure, he will often experience the appropriate bodily sensations, or else the doctor will give some other proof of the operation, such as a final scar from the incision and sutures. Mediums and their spiritual doctors are also often assisted by 'nurses' who are typically novice mediums who have not yet become proficient at performing while in possession trance, but who have 'doctors' with whom they work nonecstatically. Their treatments consist mainly of massages and medical cleansings. The following is an account of a woman's spiritual operation:

Alicia had been suffering from 'colitis' for some time, and repeatedly prayed to God to allow her to have a spiritual operation. Then one day while sitting with her eyes closed in a *cátedra* He spoke to her saying that if she truly had faith in Him, she could have the operation. Then He gave her the following instructions: 'It's going to be Wednesday at 8:00 p.m. You must get clean white sheets; the entire bed must be white, and you must have a new white smock [the kind worn by mediums at services]. Everything you put on must be white; I don't want anything coloured. And at the head of your bed, you must put a towel, a roll of bandage, a votive candle, and a spiritualist prayer book. You must also buy a bedpan because you are going to need it.' Alicia bought these items plus new white stockings and underclothes, and some cloth from which she made a new smock. Then she invited a friend, Gaspar, who is able 'to see', to come and observe the operation. On the appointed day he arrived with a medium in whom the 'doctor', named *Jorge Torre de la Tribu de David*, would appear. As the time approached, they turned out the lights and with a flashlight began to read prayers. Then Alicia lay on her bed, and soon felt the side of her abdomen being washed with a swab of cotton. 'I was conscious, but as when one thinks they are asleep, but is actually awake. They[9] allowed me "to see", such that I was observing the entire operation.' After being washed she felt an injection of anaesthetic and then saw the spiritual doctor make an incision in her side with a scalpel into which, using forceps, he inserted cotton swabs and from which he excised some body tissues. She also observed herself bleeding profusely from the incision. The operation was completed with sutures. 'And just as I saw the operation Brother Gaspar also saw it, and for this reason I had no doubt that I had in fact been operated on.' When the operation was over, the spiritual doctor spoke to her, telling her to continue lying on her back without moving. 'Then I became very hot, and when the anaesthetic wore off I felt a great pain in my waist. My father [God] put this pain in me to further show where He had operated.' The pain was severe enough to cause her to cry. On the next and subsequent days the medium returned, each time going into possession trance so that the spirit doctor could in effect make house calls on the re-cuperating patient. On the second of these calls he told her that she had to remain in bed for forty days and gave her dietary instructions to follow during this period: no greasy foods, only toasted bread, milk, and chicken soup. She remained in bed for six days virtually without moving. On the sixth day the spirit told her that she was to get up to have her bedclothes changed, which he did working through the medium. He then changed the bedding which he said was covered with blood from the operation, and then put her back into the clean bed and placed two pillows under her head, and ordered her to lie in a supine position without moving until he returned. Three days later the medium and spirit doctor returned and got Alicia up on her feet again, and told her that she was doing well and could walk about the house, if she took only half steps. When the medium again returned after several days, Alicia was having severe pains in the area of her operation and the spirit explained that this was because she was not walking as instructed, and scolded her for disobeying, ordering her back to bed and to use the bedpan for three days. When the medium returned at the end of these three days, the spirit said that Alicia was recuperated enough to go out of the house if she walked with half steps, and did not ride in automobiles or buses. According to her own account she recovered completely from the operation with virtual complete elimination of her symptoms in about three months.

It is in evocation of such strong imagery that spiritualism differs greatly from Western psychotherapy with its reliance on verbal analysis and associations. It is this capacity to bring to life images of everything from features of the spiritualist cosmology to one's own body parts, organ systems, and tissues that is its distinctive feature and therapeutic asset.

PARANOIA AND ANXIETY

The socially and economically marginal situation of many recruits to spiritualism is stressful and results in much fear and anxiety about personal security. For the most part these emotions are based on a realistic perception of their life situation, and cannot be considered neurotic in the sense that they involve delusional thought. But in many cases this constant anxiety and fear colours perceptions of the local environment in general. Collectively these attitudes become projected into folk concepts which in turn are thought of as true, or at least quite possibly true, images of reality. In the lives of spiritualists, the assumed presence of witches is the most significant of such reifications. My own rough estimate, based on nonrandomly collected case histories and on the estimates of mediums, is that in 90 per cent of all cases, witchcraft is the diagnosed cause of symptoms for which relief is sought in spiritualism. Witches are insidious in that they usually conceal their identities and attack victims surreptitiously, either from a distance by magic, or by poisoning food.

Psychologically similar to witchcraft is the widespread belief in the evil eye and the dangerous properties of the atmosphere, namely *aires,* which are believed to cause much illness.[10] These are typical of paranoid projections in general in that they are seen as malignant forces, which with little rhyme or reason may attack the relatively defenceless victim.

Thus, through the mechanism of projection, people living in a noxious and stressful situation create additional symbolic threats which, since they are taken as real, exacerbate stress and resultant anxiety. Indeed, many such individuals appear to spend more time and effort at protecting themselves and seeking cure from the effects of these reified threats than in coping with the primary stresses which generate them.

Although these forces are thought to be capable of harming one by damaging his or her property or relatives, in almost all cases the attack is assumed to be on the victim's physical and, consequently, mental well-being. These perceptions are constantly reinforced by the medical complaints endemic in the social strata from which most spiritualists are recruited. Concern with personal health can be considered mildly obsessive in perhaps 50 per cent of all spiritualists, and although Western psychiatry does not make such an association, this hypochondriasis can be seen as linked to the underlying paranoid attitude.

The spiritualist strategy for treating paranoid complaints is to deal with the senses of powerlessness and defencelessness felt in the face of superior, overwhelming, threatening forces. Working within the cosmological assumptions of spiritualism, the healer does this by marshalling positive power in the service of the patient. Here visual imagery is important: the possessed medium may describe how curative, protective forces, rays, or streams of light are showering down on the invalid. Some mediums and their patients are protected by luminous rings which circle them and through which evil spirits cannot penetrate. If the invalid is so disposed, he may 'see' these forces working on his behalf, and in all likelihood those present who are capable of 'seeing' will also confirm these things. In any event, the entry of 'forces' into mediums and 'doctors' is quite evident in that this 'energy' causes their bodies to shake and tremble.

As can be seen from the above, the tendency for delusional thought, hallucination, sense of personal inadequacy, and a concern with superhuman powers and forces characteristic of paranoia is not fundamentally changed in spiritualist therapy. Instead the contents are restructured so that the reconstituted images and assumptions are less disconcerting and the behaviour predicated on them socially more harmonious.

Socialization into this new way of thinking is facilitated by the practice of 'analysis'. Following ceremonies in most temples, all present are encouraged to describe whatever trance phenomena they experienced so that the group can collctively attempt to 'analyse' their meaning. At this time, senior adepts adroitly interpret their own and the visions and dreams of others in positive terms. They are quick to tell novices and visitors that their visions and dreams signify that they are protected by spirit-beings or have special latent powers which they must work to develop. Negative experiences in particular are interpreted to reveal some hidden positive meanings. Also, while curing the medium inevitably places her hands upon the front and back of the invalid's head so that the curative power which is concentrated in her 'enters' the invalid, who may experience this as a jolt of power, while the possessed medium repeats phrases such as *yo te fortalesco* (I am fortifying you). The intensity with which the medium clasps her hands on the invalid's head causes him to tremble, heightening the effect that the electrical-like power of the spirit-being is passing into his head and body. The healer is thus seen as a conduit or repository of positive forces, and this assumption is supported by the constant reiteration that spiritualism is entirely positive: it is associated with daylight, the colour white, and benevolent spirit-beings, as opposed to witchcraft and evil in general, which are associated with nighttime, darkness, and the devil.

The malignant influences which are displaced from the patient by the positive forces radiating from the medium are often conceptualized as flowing, at least in part, into her, as though she had in effect established a two-way channel between herself and the patient. Therefore, after treating severely ill individuals, the healer must subsequently divest herself of whatever substance she has absorbed from the patient. She does this while staggering about with pains in her head and body, by repeatedly stroking herself, 'cleansing' herself and 'throwing away' the accumulated poison or evil influence. This transfer of the sickness to the healer is further dramatic evidence to the patient that he has truly been divested of it.

Several basic preventive and healing practices – especially magical protection from harmful forces and ritual purification – are conceptually related to the great concern with magical attack and poisoning. The most widely used technique in spiritualist healing, borrowed from traditional Mexican folk medicine, is the *limpia,* or cleansing. Cleansing may be done merely by stroking the body, either one's own or someone else's, as described above. Flowers and especially whisks of the California pepper tree, the *pirul (Shinus molle)* also serve well for this. The widespread use of the pirul and its semi-sacred status are no doubt due to the pungency of its foliage, as is also true of the cleansing herbs rue and rosemary. Other sharp-smelling substances are similarly opposed to maligant forces. Thus, dilute solutions of ammonia water are rubbed over one's clothing and head before entering temples, and in some temples everyone present is first cleansed with billows of smoke produced by sprinkling a combination of *copal* (resins from the trees of the family *Burseraceae*) and church incense onto burning charcoal. The visibility and pungency of the smoke, the pungency of pirul, and the fragrance of flowers and perfume, which are also used for 'protection', all have in common properties perceptible to human senses. At the same time they are ethereal substances similar to the invisible malignancies which pervade the atmosphere. But subject to human control, they can thus be used to displace and fend off the invisible influences. Another instance of this is the use of water and vegetable oils which are left in open containers on or near the altars in temples so that they can accumulate the positive forces that 'descend' there. The preventative and curative effects of perfumes and flowers are also enhanced in this way. This 'holy water' is taken home where it serves primarily to absorb evil influences penetrating one's house. A glass of it is left above the door, or a bottle of it is placed under the bed for a few days and then disposed of ritually. Here the water acts to absorb rather than displace. It is also frequently drunk, and in this case its presumed therapeutic action is less evident. The oils are used for anointing and massaging.

The logical relationships between malignant forces and the curative properties of water and other things such as flowers, perfume, as well as the possessed healing medium is unclear, or possibly simply inconsistent. On the one hand the curative substances are effective because they are charged with positive forces which usually dispel malignant ones, while on the other they also have an absorbent quality. Although it is difficult to quantify such things, it is apparent that far greater use is made of the displacive actions of magical substances than their absorbent qualities. This folk model is consistent with an image of the world in which processes and phenomena in general are the result of interacting, opposed dynamic forces. Normalcy, both in terms of health and social relations, is seen as a state of equilibrium between such forces.

These interactions of positive and malevolent forces in spiritualist cosmology are a replication of a fundamental principle of dynamism in traditional Mexican thought which is most explicitly expressed in the concepts of 'hot' and 'cold', derived from classical Greek natural history and brought to Mexico via sixteenth-century Spain. In their present form in contemporary Mexican folk medicine, 'heat' and 'cold' are abstract qualities inherent in various quantities in all material and many immaterial phenomena. Accordingly, aspects of the natural world, especially foods, remedies and emotions, are so classified, usually on a three- or four-point scale of relative hotness to coldness. Health depends on having proper amounts of both qualities. If one is exposed to excessive quantities of one or the other it displaces or absorbs its counterpart, resulting in sickness. In spiritualism concern with hot and cold is attenuated, but the underlying dualism is firmly intact. Thus, the chief concern is not with heat and cold *per se*, but rather the interaction of less specific, and in many ways more awesome, forces.

A final and not insignificant benefit that paranoid individuals derive from participation in spiritualism is entry into a group of friendly, warm, supportive people, whose presence, reinforced by the positive powers, to some extent offsets obsessive or near obsessive concern with a pseudo-community of witches. We will return to this communal aspect of therapy below.

DEPRESSION

The marginality and insecurity in which most adepts live results in many complaints of general mental and physical malaise which can be summed up as depression. These symptoms typically include insomnia, lack of energy, loneliness, uncontrollable weeping, and anxiety.

The most immediate anti-depressive aspect of spiritualist events and officiating personnel is, as in the case of paranoia, the 'energy' or 'forces' that they bring to the service of the individual. But here this energy serves not, as in the case of the paranoid, to displace malevolent forces, but rather to infuse and energize the depressed person. At the beginning of a service, the general mood is typically subdued and melancholic. As participants start gathering, those who are depressed often sit apart, bent over, sometimes weeping, As the service progresses, the ecstatic experiences of mediums are often contagious, and non-mediums may spontaneously go into less intense states of dissociation, sometimes accompanied by glossolalia or other ecstatic speech. Simultaneously, other participants may animatedly describe visions that they are experiencing. But one need not have such experiences to benefit from them, 'to feel the force enter your body'. The atmosphere becomes electric, and one feels that one is participating in extraordinary events. The collective mood, which at the beginning of the service is subdued if not maudlin, is at the end animated and even effervescent.

The sense of belonging to a friendly group which helps to allay paranoia is also effective against the symptoms of depression in the following way. Just as membership in spiritualism provides a positive social circle for paranoids assaulted by insidious forces and persons, it also becomes a surrogate family for those who have few or no immediate relatives or others able to provide security. This new family is largely a symbolic creation elaborated in patterns of speech and behaviour. Most obvious here is the use of the term *hermano* (sibling) for all human participants in the cult. It is also interesting, though no doubt accidental, that the mediums are referred to as *materias,* a term etymologically related to 'mother', for while in possession trance they relate to their 'children' in a very maternal, nurturing manner. The more revered mediums are typically stout, post-menopausal women who assume a posture in possession trance which expresses a profound, unshakeable strength and solidity. The positive spirits possessing a medium address the followers with such terms as *niños amados* (beloved children), *mi hija* (my daughter), or *tú de mi pequeña* (my little one). Whether an adept approaches the possessed medium voluntarily or is summoned in front of her by a possessing spirit, the exchange is highly charged emotionally, with the adept often breaking into sobs or profuse sweating while requesting some favour or fervently thanking the possessing spirit. The adept's speech is apt to deteriorate somewhat here, as though the situation allows her to become more child-like under the benevolent protection of the medium-spirit.

This emotional regression itself serves to enhance the distinction between the bent, sobbing 'child' and the erect, all-loving, protective, nurturing medium-spirit. In this guise the medium shares common features with the Virgin Mary of Mexican folk Catholicism. But whereas a major feature of the Virgin is her capacity for suffering and her mediating position between her supplicants and God, the medium in effect *is* God in that He or a refraction – a symbolic equivalent – of Him, such as Father Elijah or Father Jesus, has entered into her. Whereas the cult of the Virgin can be seen as a projection of the *mestizo* family in which children, especially sons, relate to psychologically and socially absent patriarchal fathers through the mother-wife,[11] within the symbolic spiritualist family the absent father returns in positive form by means of the medium. The maternal female medium possessed by a benevolent omnipotent male spirit is thus an androgynous figure which, in one stroke, becomes the loving, protective, healing parent to a group of abandoned, lonely, suffering 'children'. The ideal family circle of powerful, compassionate parents and many loving children – 'brothers' and 'sisters' – is thus complete.

Not only does spiritualism relate to the superficial symptoms of depression as just discussed, but for those prone to possession trance it also provides a context and means by which introjected hostility, if present, can be mobilized and expressed outwardly through legitimized catharsis. The following incident illustrates this:

Fifteen mediums were simultaneously in possession trance, working together in the ceremony called 'passing beings to the light', in which each medium lends her body temporarily to one spirit of a deceased person after another so that these spirits may have the benefit of the light of day which will enhance their chances of finding peace. Then one of the mediums announced that some soldiers who had been killed during the Revolution were going to appear. Another of the mediums who was also 'working' came out of trance at this point, and since she has the power of *videncia*, she observed what then ensued, describing it to the many non-visionaries who were attending the ceremony. What follows is a synopsis of her account, which essentially agrees with other accounts told to me independently by other witnesses. Two bands of guerrillas appeared, one led by Pancho Villa, the other by some other general. Soldiers from the two respective bands then began to enter into the enraptured mediums so that they could use their bodies to resume a battle that had been terminated by their deaths, which they immediately began to do, much to the consternation of the many people who were in the temple. The non-visionaries saw only the two groups of mediums locked in combat – wrestling on the floor, scratching, kicking, and pummelling each other. Those visionaries who also had the power of 'hearing' heard the sounds of the invisible pistols, rifles, and machine guns that the soldiers were firing. Eventually some of the noncombatants who were present were able to dispel the possessing spirits from the tussling mediums in the standard way – directing, by word and gesture, 'light and progress' onto them. When the spirits of the soldiers departed, the mediums 'awoke', and after the event was told to them, they then bandaged their real abrasions and contusions, and also cured various 'invisible' wounds that they had inflicted on one another.

The actions of 'bad' possessing spirits are usually less dramatic, being confined for the most part to the use of lascivious language. Well-established mediums do not often engage in such behaviour, but it is a way in which individuals prone to possession trance can benignly act out repressed impulses and emotions which are otherwise inappropriate to express. Such catharsis also no doubt serves as a built-in safety valve to minimize personal frictions that build up among individuals congregating in a particular temple. One common type of conflict results from competition among budding mediums for the favour of the major medium of a temple. Tensions also develop between advanced mediums and their apprentices as the latter begin to become mediums in their own right. Invidious comparison and competition for the allegiance of adepts inevitably ensues and eventually causes apprentices who are determined to become independent mediums to break with their mentors and establish temples of their own. In the absence of central authority

and an organized hierarchy responsible for the growth of spiritualism, these mini-schisms are the principal way in which it
spreads in the general population.

Possession Trance and Personal Change

Not only novice spiritualists, but mediums themselves benefit from
the appearance of spirits and powers. Most immediately they reap
financial benefits. Although they are enjoined by principle to not
charge for healing, they readily accept 'donations'. The more
successful mediums thus gain financial independence and this in
itself is a strong inducement to practise their art, and is also of no
small therapeutic value in providing a measure of material security. Mediums also obtain psychological benefits from repeatedly
experiencing culturally appropriate possession trance. One is the
immediate transformation in personality that the trancer under-
goes during possession. The performance allows for the acting out
of repressed desires and impulses, and also for the assumption of
different identities. This alteration of identity is temporary, lasting
only for the period of the possession, but the dissociation experience
and the social performance also influence the medium's general
non-trance identity. Although the actual possession phase of a performance is not remembered, the entry into and coming out of
possession trance are recalled. The induction phase in particular is
often intensely experienced. This is frequently described as being
'inflated': 'I feel as though I am becoming larger, as though my
bosom, my chest is swelling up.' (This sensation may be influenced
by the strong rising and falling of the chest due to the deep breathing that is carried out during trance induction.) After coming out
of a positive possession trance mediums report a deep sense of
expansion and contentment which lingers on as an afterglow,
markedly colouring their general state of being. In addition to this
psychological change experienced by the medium, she also
acquires a new social status. She becomes defined as a semi-sacred
person within her social setting by virtue of being a vehicle for the
manifestation of renowned spirits. In other words, her new identity
is validated and reinforced by the approbation given to it by the
adepts who venerate her. For spiritualist healers who are not capable of full possession trance, the title 'doctor' is a mark of increased

personal prestige and status comparable to that acquired by
mediums.

One final aspect which bears on the identity of the medium
needs to be examined, and this is the relationship that is formed
between her and the spirits that possess her. From a Durkheimian
perspective one would expect that the spirit world would in some
way replicate the human world. But instead, as we saw above, the
sociology of the divine is essentially an inversion of the human:
whereas the bulk of adepts recruited to spiritualism are relatively
powerless women, the spirits who take an interest in them are, with
few exceptions, powerful males. I have described above the various
paramount 'father' spirits that occupy the central positions within
the spiritualist pantheon. In terms of frequency of appearance in
possession trance and as visionary experiences, spiritual doctors are
the next most significant beings after refractions of the 'father'. Of
fifteen spiritual doctors on which I have information, all are male.
Interestingly, these healing 'doctors' are all exotic characters –
Japanese, Black, Indian, Hebrew, etc.

For the relatively non-ecstatic spiritualist, i.e. an adept who is
prone to trance states, but not to possession trance, the spirits who
appear to them via mediums can be seen as momentary and symbolic replacements for the husbands and fathers they lack. But the
situation is quite different for the mediums in whom these spirits
appear. For here the identity of the medium versus that of the
possessing spirit is not so clear. While the medium is 'working', her
spirit is believed to depart from her body under the care of her
protector so that the possessing spirit may come into it. But in spite
of this distinction between the soul of the medium and the visiting
spirit, the identity of the medium vis-à-vis the in-dwelling spirit is
complex. In one sense the medium has merely lent her body to the
spirit but in another sense she has temporarily become that spirit;
the boundaries between the two become blurred. Spiritualists
occasionally reveal this confusion by inappropriately referring to
a male possessing spirit as 'she'. It is by virtue of this intimate
association with revered spirits that mediums come to occupy the
most esteemed positions within spiritualism. Prior to taking up this
ecstatic vocation they are typically socially isolated, 'abandoned'
women; as mediums they, in a very real sense, come to acquire not
only the financial but also the social identity that is otherwise more
typically a prerogative of the men of the communities, as epitom-

ized in the masculine spirits which possess them.

The one major exception to this taking on of forceful male roles in possession trance is the occasional appearance, in several peripheral mediums, of the Virgin Mary, the fourth of the Divinities. As in the case of possession by the male spirit-beings, here again there is assimilation of sacred status to personal identity, with attendant symbolic and social gains. A reason for selection of this particular feminine role, rather than a powerful male role more characteristic of the mediumistic repertoire is suggested by the following psychiatric case of a delusional Mexican-American woman who believed that she was the Virgin Mary, 'a common theme among Mexican-American women with psychotic illnesses'.[12]

> Her life had been hard and she felt she had sinned against God. She became increasingly depressed, anxious and self accusatory and could not function adequately in her role of wife and mother until she heard the voice of God speaking to her. From this experience, she became convinced that she was the Virgin Mary, a delusional idea the acceptance of which served to reduce her anxiety and distress by providing her with an explanation (albeit false) of her experience.[13]

By taking on this role, not only is the medium's suffering explained and validated to her, but she becomes exalted in the eyes of others, which is a further compensation.

Summary

The essential features of spiritualist therapy are its ability to evoke powerful imagery, especially of body parts and aspects of the spiritual cosmology, and to loosen blocked emotions. Powerful suggestions, experienced as visualization of body ailments and their magical treatment, serve to remove many symptoms, especially those of a hysterical nature, and are also no doubt quite effective in generally mobilizing natural healing potentials.

As for paranoid delusions, which are remarkably resistant to rational explanation, ecstatic experiences or the infectious ecstacy of the enraptured mediums provide the paranoid with experiential demonstration of powerful supernatural forces working on his or her behalf. Similarly, it is arousal of such ecstasy or near ecstasy which dispels the melancholia of the depressed. In all cases, spiritualist therapy is possible because patients and healers have the same magical, animistic vision of the world, a world view which is both engendered and perpetuated by the spiritualist cosmology and experiences. Finally, mediums themselves reap considerable personal benefit from the practice of their art. In addition to financial rewards, they acquire new personal identities by repeated entry into sacred ecstatic states and by merging their own selves with those of powerful, revered supernatural beings.

NOTES AND REFERENCES

1   I wish to thank those who read and commented on an earlier version of this paper: Spencer Kagan, Isabel Kelly, Carole Nagengast, Paul Rosenblatt, James Stuart, and Anna Garcia who also assisted me during part of the field work. This research was supported by intramural grants from the University of California, Riverside.

2   'Spiritualism' (*espiritualismo*) is used throughout this paper since it is the term that my informants apply to themselves. For a discussion of the ethnographic status of spiritualism-spiritism in Mexico and among Mexican-Americans, see J. Macklin, 'Folk saints, healers, and spiritist cults in Northern Mexico', *Revista Interamericano Review*, Vol. 3, No. 4, Winter 1974, pp. 351-67.

3   For additional discussion of its origin and ethnography elsewhere in Mexico see M. Kearney, 'Espiritualismo as an alternative medical tradition in the border area', to appear in *Modern Medicine and Medical Anthropology in the Border Population*, Pan American Health Organization; idem, 'Oral performance by Mexican spiritualists in possession trance', to appear in the *Journal of Latin American Lore;* I. Kelly, 'Mexican spiritualism', *Kroeber Anthropological Society Papers,* No. 25, Fall 1961, pp. 191-206; idem, *Folk Practices in North Mexico,* Austin, University of Texas Press, 1965; I. Lagarriga Attias, *Medicina Tradicional y Espiritismo,* Mexico, Secretaria de Educacion Publica, 1975; J. Macklin, op. cit.; idem, 'Belief, ritual, and healing: New England spiritualism and Mexican-American spiritism compared', in Zaretsky and Leone (eds.), *Religious Movements in Contemporary America,* Princeton, Princeton University Press, 1974, pp. 383-417; idem, 'Santo folk, curanderismo y cults espiritistas en Mexico: eleccion divina y seleccion social', *Annuario Indigenista,* Vol. 34, December 1974, pp. 195-214.

4   John A. Price, *Tijuana: Urbanization in a Border Culture,* Notre Dame, Indiana, University of Notre Dame Press, 1973.

5   Nelson attributes the rise of spiritualism in the eastern United States in the late 1800s to conditions similar to those in Baja California: frontier atmosphere, increased anomie due to chaotic cultural patterns resulting from high immigration rate of diverse national groups, and rapid industrialization. Geoffrey Nelson, *Spiritualism and Society,* New York, Schocken, 1969.

6   E. Bourguignon, 'Introduction: a framework for the comparative study of altered states of consciousness', in E. Bourguignon (ed.), *Religion, Altered States of Consciousness, and Social Change,* Columbus, Ohio, Ohio State University Press, 1973, pp. 3-35.

7   For a discussion of this and relevant citations see Martin Seligman, *Helplessness: On Depression, Development, and Death,* San Francisco, Freeman & Co., 1975, pp. 167-88.

8   See, for example, P. Lowinger and S. Dobie, 'What makes the placebo work?', *Archives of General Psychiatry,* Vol. 20, January 1969, pp. 84-8; Jerome Frank, Chapter 6, 'The placebo effect and the role of expectations in medical and psychological treatment', in *Persuasion and Healing,* Baltimore, The Johns Hopkins University Press, 1973, pp. 136-64.

9   Reference to a possessing spirit is often in the third person plural.

10   For further discussion and analysis of the paranoid psychology of the evil eye, *aires,* and witchcraft see M. Kearney, *The Winds of Ixtepeji: World View and Society in a Zapotec Town,* New York, Holt, Rinehart and Winston, 1972, pp. 46-58; idem, 'A world view explanation of the evil eye', in C. Maloney (ed.), *The Evil Eye,* New York, Columbia University Press, 1974, pp. 175-92.

11   E. R. Wolf, 'The Virgin of Guadalupe: a Mexican national symbol', *Journal of American Folklore,* Vol. 71, No. 279, January-March 1958, pp. 34-9.

12   Ari Kiev, *Curanderismo: Mexican-American Folk Psychiatry,* New York, The Free Press, 1968.

13   Ibid.

Barbara Kerewsky Halpern and John Miles Foley

3

Bajanje: Healing Magic in Rural Serbia

In traditional cultures some of the most important forms of ritual
were those which served to mediate between events 'here' in this
world and those seen as coming from 'out of there', from the nether
world. The skills of the practitioners – magicians, conjurers and
sorcerers – effected cures, worked protective and sometimes evil
magic, and exercised control over a range of wordly and other-
wordly relationships. The ritual performer could be priest, healer,
and judge. His utterances took the form of charms, spells, incantations, and supplications and have been viewed by some scholars as
analogous to prayer.[1]

As part of an ongoing study of aspects of oral tradition in the
Balkans[2] in this paper we present evidence that healing charms are
still being transmitted orally and continue as part of the contemporary folk repertoire. Our concern here is with process, both
cultural and linguistic. We want to discover why as well as how
orality works as a vital means of preservation and transmission.

This we undertake by examing *bajanje,* a form of folk curing
relying primarily on incantation. Texts of *basme,* oral charms
uttered by practitioners of this type of medicine, have been
reported by local ethnographers and others over the past fifty
years.[3] While these fragments are of interest comparatively, in
order to demonstrate oral process it is necessary to work from an
inventory of 'complete' texts of a particular charm.[4] Towards this
end we have based analysis on our recent field recordings made in
Serbia, backed by extensive prior research in the same geographical
area.[5]

40

In the present study we first describe the cultural setting in which such charms are found. A representative *basma* is given in translation. (The Serbo-Croation text, as recorded during the course of field work, appears in an Appendix.)[6] A structural analysis is then made on several levels, isolating internal frames and examining linguistic and symbolic components.[7] Diagrammatic representation of symbolic action shows how the *bajanje* functions spatially and temporally to effect the cure through the mediation of the *bajalica* (conjuror).

The Setting

The region of Sumadija in central Serbia is characterized by ethnic homogeneity. Originally wooded, it later supported a peasant subsistence economy based on a combination of herding and mixed cultivation, a pattern consistent with the needs of the multi-generational South Slav extended family household. Ancestors of today's population began to migrate into the area towards the end of the eighteenth century, when Turkish control was on the wane in that part of the Balkans. From their mountain homeland in Montenegro they brought with them a highly structured patri-archal and patrilocal social order and a proud identity defined and refined by oral tradition – by the performance of epics of medieval Serbian heroes from the time of the Turkish conquest and earlier, by the sense of self in the recollection of genealogies back to the founders of lineages, and by the practical wisdom exemplified in *narodni lek* (folk medicine).[8]

In many respects the extended household was a largely self-sufficient unit, providing from within for most of the economic, physical, and emotional needs of its members. Some men were part-time tanners, carpenters, or distillers. Any elder with a *gusle*, the single-stringed instrument used to accompany the singing of heroic epics, could be a bard. Some women were skilled in dyeing and weaving, or in healing with herbs and grasses. In Sumadija formal religion was never crucial in shaping attitudes; being a Serb meant being a member of the Serbian Orthodox faith. The head of the household was in a sense his own priest, personally conducting the most important ritual occasion of the yearly cycle, the *slava* ceremony honouring his clan's patron saint. He was on comfortable terms with God, interceding directly on behalf of the entire family.

It was not the function of this patriarchal and collective structure, however, to deal with magic and devilry, to banish diseases caused by mysterious chthonic powers, to counteract the evil eye, to divine, to bewitch. For this work specialists were required; their activities were self-directed and free from customary responsibilities to the group. Some performed magic mainly by means of ritual objects (*vracanje*). Others mediated mainly with the power of words, and it is this *bajanje* which we will examine.

In rural Serbia today, as in contemporary Yugoslavia generally, with the increasing participation of peasants in the cash economy of an industrializing socialist nation, traditional patterns are undergoing marked changes of all kinds. The regional market town now provides most peasant needs, including the services of doctors and pharmacists. 'But,' says one man, 'for some things, what do doctors know? Injections, injections – and nothing! For some things, *treba da se baje* [you have to cure with charms].'

, People say that folk magic is now legally forbidden. However, with the tradition of secrecy surrounding these skills and the state's tolerance for limited, small-scale private enterprise, divining and conjuring do persist in the villages. These practices maintain a continuity of services in response to individual needs. In addition, there is continuity in the traditional oral transmission of such specialized knowledge. In Serbia, as in most parts of the Balkans, practitioners have been women exclusively.[9] This sex distinction is still manifest in the allocation of ritual roles: within the conventions of society, the regularized cycle of ritual acts remains primarily the province of men; non-regularized, secret activities are the domain of females.

Charms are regarded as an inheritance, items of great usefulness to be preserved and passed on. Young girls are taught these *basme* by their mothers or grandmothers, and they may also be present while a grandmother is actually performing. An in-marrying bride can learn from her mother-in-law or grandmother-in-law.[10] This is how a woman in her sixties recalls acquiring a charm from her grandmother some fifty-five years ago: '*Baba* told me, 'Go sit in the corner, child, and pay attention!' So I did. Later she told me what the whispering and mumbling meant. She taught me, so I learned it and remembered it, and that's how I know how to say it.' A woman now in her mid-forties describes her experience: 'When I was preparing to marry, my mother gave me this [charm] and she said, "This is nice for you to have, daughter. With it you can help others. It will be *sevap* [a good deed]." Thus I received it. And now,' she adds, 'I can use it.' Unbroken lines of transmission, whether consanguineal or affinal, are felt by villagers to be important,[11] and practitioners pass their special knowledge on to selected receivers only.[12]

While a female of any age may learn a charm, only a ritually clean (i.e. post-menstrual) woman may actively practise *bajanje*. This convention designates a time span of up to thirty-five years or so during which she is restricted from performing the charm. It thus places her within the ancient and widespread belief system in which females of child-bearing age are defined as a special class, in possession of dual powers, one sacred and related to the cyclical properties so similar to the mysteries of nature, and the other polluting and negative.[13] Both aspects are seen as potentially dangerous, a fact articulated even by contemporary villagers. Another consideration, particularly within the structure of a strongly patriarchal society, is that during these years a woman is viewed as part of a procreative unit and not as an individual (in many parts of the Balkans, upon marriage a bride's given name is dropped, and her first name becomes the possessive inflected form of her husband's). Only menopausal women, therefore, are non-threatening as mediators with the nether world. At the same time, the effectiveness of old women as healers draws on their experience in traditional female roles as nurturers and protectors.

Despite occasional reinforcement by hearing the charm and perhaps even transmitting it, the prescribed period of restriction on actual *bajanje* raises interesting questions with regard to retention.[14] A linguistic analysis of the *basma* presented below would isolate those features which serve to trigger recall. These include larger thematic and structural components, the connective links between them, and the smaller, more subtle factors of assonance and stress. The language of the charm and the societal motivation to preserve and transmit it, functioning within a still largely traditional oral culture, share in accounting for the ability to recollect without active use over so long a time in a woman's life.

The Conjurer Desanka

Against this background we now introduce Desanka, a practising
bajalica. She is a robust, pleasant-looking woman of fifty-seven.
Unlike most village women of that age, she goes about her household work with her head uncovered. Were it not for her calloused
hands and bare feet, Desanka would resemble an urban matron.
From her appearance, so unlike that of the stereotype of the
wrinkled Balkan crone peering out from the folds of a dark ker-
chief, one would not surmise that she is a conjurer of considerable
local repute. She is the eldest female in a four-generation household of which her aged, widowed father-in law is the titular head.
The other members are her husband and their elder son, daughter-
in-law, and two grandchildren. Their younger son is a factory
worker in Germany, and Desanka has been to visit him there. He
took her to a doctor to treat her recurrent arthritis. 'Their aspirin
is better than ours,' she maintains.

Desanka is recognized as a specialist in dealing with diseases
called the 'nine winds'. Villagers perceive these illnesses as both
borne on and caused by the powers of the wind (*vetar*). Although
the terminology involved is no longer part of the contemporary
lexicon, a classificatory system of winds persists, assigning qualities
('sprightly', 'gusty', and so forth) and designating colours as syn-
onymous with a perceived class of skin disorders. For example,
they call erysipelas the 'red wind', eczema the 'white wind', and
anthrax the 'black wind'.

When we stopped by to visit (on 30 July, 1975), Desanka was
pasturing pigs. Following traditions of hospitality, she ushered us
inside the whitewashed, mud-brick house and offered ritual serv-
ings of *slatko* (sweet preserves), homemade brandy, and Turkish
coffee. Eventually, reassured by the presence of her husband, who
had come in from the hay field, she raced through a recitation of
the charm to dispel the red wind (*crveni vetar*). When she hesitated
at one point in this first performance, her seven-year-old grandson
Marko prompted her.[15] The resultant uneven pace provided a
logical reason to ask Desanka to repeat the *basma*. A third version
was elicited by asking for clarification of a certain passage; in order
to retrieve that small section, she had to go back and start from the
beginning.

After making a preliminary analysis of three charm variants, we returned to Desanka eight days later, explaining that some of the archaic language was unfamiliar to us. In this manner we came to understand better the folk interpretations of the role of the *bajalica* as mediator. Her comments also revealed much about village attitudes towards psychic healing, notions of wind-borne diseases, and the dynamics of transmission. During this second session we obtained on tape five additional versions of the same charm. Her daughter-in-law Nada was present most of the time, and towards the end of the visit she suggested fetching Desanka's *pribor* (equipment), so that they could re-enact a 'real' cure, with Nada in the role of the afflicted person kneeling before the conjurer. The result was an irregular text of the charm, a situation recognized by Desanka herself, preoccupied as she was with illustrating the use of the conjuring tools (feather, knife, stone, and coal scuttle with a live ember). Conscious of enunciating for the tape recorder, she explained that she was not accustomed to thinking of the words: 'When I'm saying it for real, it's like whispering. I recall the words, and what I don't recall I dream at night.'

The Charm[16]

(a) 1. Out of there comes the red horse,
  2. The red man, the red mouth,
  3. The red arms, the red legs,
  4. The red mane, the red hooves.

(b) 5. As he comes, so he approaches,
  6. He lifts out the disease immediately;

(c) 7. He carries it off and carries it away,
  8. Across the sea without delay –

(d) 9. Where the cat doesn't meow,
  10. Where the pig doesn't grunt,
  11. Where the sheep don't bleat,
  12. Where the goats don't low,

(e)   13. Where the priest doesn't come,
     14. Where the cross isn't borne,
     15. So that ritual bread isn't broken,
     16. So that candles aren't lit.

(f)   17. Banish the disease into the field,
     18. Banish the disease into the sea,
     19. Banish the disease under a stone;
     20. You have no place here!

(g)   21. Out of there comes the red cow,
     22. She bore a red calf,
     23. She provided red milk.

(h)   24. Out of there comes the red hen,
     25. She leads nine red chicks,
     26. She fell upon a red dung heap,
     27. She gathered up red worms.

(c)   28. And she carried [it] off across the sea,
     29. Across the sea without delay.

(f)   30. Banish the illness into the field,
     31. Banish the illness into the sea,
     32. Banish the illness;
     33. You have no place here!

(i)   — Let [name] remain
     34. Light[ly] as a feather,
     35. Pure as silver,
     36. Mild as mother's milk.

(j)   37. Out of there comes Ugimir,
     38. Kill the disease, kill it!
     39. Out of there comes Stanimir,
     40. Halt the disease, halt it!
     41. Out of there comes Persa,
     42. Stop the disease, stop it!

(k)   43. Ten, nine, eight, seven,
      44. Six, five, four, three, two, one.

(l)   45. Into the wolf's legs, and the fifth, the tail.
      46. Out of my speaking has come the cure! [17]

In order to accomplish that removal, she summons a series of exorcizing agents, all of whom are introduced by the 'Out of there comes the (named agent) *Otud ide*/name' formula, echoing the opening line of the charm. The first three in this pattern – the horse and rider, the cow, and the hen – are also conjured according to colour; that is, they are suited in both nature and origin to the task they are to undertake.[18] Ugimir, Stanimir, and Persa also belong to the anti-world, the locus of illness, and they provide metonymic aid to the *bajalica*. The general movement of the charm, then, the return of the diseased person to his original healthy state, is twofold: (1) agents to match the disease are summoned to the natural world, and (2) these agents and the *vetar* to which they are adapted are collectively dispelled back to their common place of origin. The result is a restoration of 'here' and 'there' order, a cure which re-establishes the phenomenological balance between the two worlds.[19] The diagram below illustrates the dynamics of the exorcism process.

Situation	Element	Locus Natural World v. Anti-World
Diseased State	*vetar* (red wind)	←———————— (Intrusion of disease)
Cure, Step 1	horse and rider (a) cow (g) hen (h) symbolic names (j)	←———————— ←———————— ←———————— ←———————— (Summoning of agents)
Cure, Step 2	*vetar* (a), (g), (h), (j)	————————→ ————————→ (Banishment of disease)
Cure, Step 3	*kurjak* (wolf) (l)	←———————— (Restoration of order)

AGENTS AND THEIR FUNCTION

Symbolic Dynamics

By means of her ritual words, the *bajalica* seeks to exorcize disease. The initial situation is this: an illness from the anti-world (denoted by *otud*, 'out of there') has intruded upon the natural world (denoted by *tu*, 'here') and has become a destructive force that challenges the normal order. Were it still located in that 'other' place, 'where the cat doesn't meow', all would be as it should and there would be no call for the restorative power of *bajanje*. But with the natural world disrupted by the presence of *crveni vetar*, more specifically with the patient suffering from erysipelas, the intercession of the conjuror is required. As a mediator between the two worlds, she will serve as a catalyst to effect a reversal of the intrusive process; that is, by means of her *odgovor* Desanka will remove the disease and consign it to its proper and orginal domain – the anti-world. The four agents assist the conjurer in various ways. The cow (g) and hen (h) are mimetic types of the *bajalica* herself, nurturing their young and affirming the continuity of the natural world. All three actions are based on a common paradigm:

X₁	provides	X₂	to nurture	X₃
cow		milk		calf
hen		worms		chicks
bajalica		*bajanje*		patient

This structural relationship sets up some important associations and oppositions that can be conveniently schematized in binary notation, with redness indicated by a plus ($+$) and lack of redness by a minus ($-$) symbol.

X₁	provides	X₂	to nurture	X₃
$+$		$+$		$+$
$+$		$+$		$+$
$-$		$-$		$+ \rightarrow -$

The cow and hen agents, though inhabitants of the anti-world ($+$), fulfil natural functions in bearing and contributing to the healthy growth of their progeny ($+$). For them it is fitting that redness be cultivated and maintained in those assigned to their care. But the patient, who lives in this world ($-$), experiences redness as a disease, a destructive influence which threatens his health. His cure involves the seeking of an appropriate maternal figure, the *bajalica* ($-$), who can provide the proper sustenance, *bajanje* ($-$), to cast out the disease ($+$) and return him to a healthy condition ($-$). Though the three actualizations of the nurturing paradigm differ with respect to the $\pm$ character of their principal elements, in each case the process is consistent in its dynamics and outcome.

The conjurer also summons first the horse and rider (a) and later the symbolic names (j) to help bring about the restoration of the order. The man on horseback comes to actively dispel the illness and carry it 'across the sea without delay' to the anti-world [(a) and (b)]. Probably a mythic figure cognate with the heroes of epic tradition, he imitates the passage of the sun through the diurnal cycle. The pattern of his journey coincides, for example, with that of a legendary figure who braved the darkness of the other world: 'And he bears himself over level Kosovo, / Even then the sun began to shine through the darkness.'[20] Like the cow and the hen, the man on horseback personifies a natural process in terms of that 'other' place, for his identity is + redness to match the disease he must bring back. In following an archetypal paradigm, he too becomes a type of *bajalica,* restoring to wholeness and order that which has been disrupted by *crveni vetar.* Appropriately, then, the (a) frame initializes the charm through the *'Otud ide* (name)' formula and the horse and rider's imitation of diurnal rhythm.[21]

The symbolic names, on the other hand, employ a somewhat different mode of mimetic exorcism. As mentioned above, Ugimir, Stanimir, and Persa contain morphemes suggestive of the verbs to 'kill', 'halt', and 'stop', respectively. If such homonymic agreement were nothing more than a series of clever collocations, we might easily dismiss this particular frame without further comment. But the three couplets, as simple as they seem, reveal the dynamics of *bajanje* at the most basic level. For behind the juxtaposition of similar syllables and the repetition of syntactic paradigms lies a belief in the power of the word, a conviction that the ultimate curative is sound articulated in a ritually prescribed manner.

The final two lines of the *basma* consistently serve as the formal termination to the ritual process. The *bajalica* sends the disease away 'into the wolf's four legs, and fifth to the tail'. The *kurjak* (wolf), co-mediator with the conjurer, acts as a passageway between the two worlds, a channel through which the *vetar* is returned from the 'here' to the 'there'.

As is forcefully illustrated in the sketch below, by a Serbian folk artist, the wolf receives the disease into his body and by this means will transfer it irreversibly across the chasm separating the natural world and the anti-world. He will deposit the disease in the anti-world, thereby restoring health, or order, to the natural world. This concept of the animal as an interface is preserved in the protective ritual of passing a newborn child through a wolf's jawbones and back out again, thus symbolically presenting the infant to the demons of the other world and returning it to safety.[23] Structurally, that return fulfils the same pattern that underlies the journey of the horse and rider and the healing art of *bajanje* itself. In the assonating last line the conjurer designates the cure as the result of her *odgovor*; by means of of its dual connotation of 'speaking out'

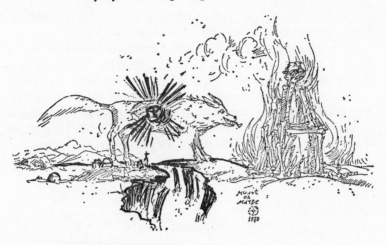

DRAWING AFTER MILIC OD MACVE [22]

and 'participation (responsibility)', this term acknowledges her role as mediator between the two worlds and as the immediate source of the charm's magic.

Transmission and Process

Unlike other genres in the oral repertoire of rural Serbia, charms are transmitted through female lines. In a patrilocal society, by the time a female is ready to pass her knowledge on to another, she has long since taken up residence away from her household of origin and thus from the *bajalica* who taught her. With the exception of affinal transmission, those who will in turn receive the charm from her will eventually move out. Over generations, then, a given *basma* is subject to transmission from family to family and place to place.

Just as it is not possible to pinpoint the geographical origins of charms, neither can we date them. Components in any synchronic recitation may include mythic symbols (the horse and rider) and Christian symbols (the priest, cross, etc.), as well as some based on relatively recent cultural adaptations, such as animal husbandry (the domesticated cow) compared to predominant pastoralism. The diachronic nature of oral process manifests itself in the combination of these kinds of elements. Oral composition has sometimes been characterized as a patchwork based on a reassembling of available parts. In fact, it is much more complex: each performance, each act of recollection, results in a new composition. The fundamental truth of the charm, and the source of its phenomenological power, lies in the ritual act of making the collective wisdom of the past the living inheritance of the present.

APPENDIX [24]

(a) 1. *Otud ide crveni konj,*
     2. *Crveni covek, crvena usta,*
     3. *Crvene ruke, crvene noge,*
     4. *Crvene grifa, crvene kopita.*

(b) 5. *Kako dodje, tako stize,*
     6. *Ovu boljku odmah dize,*

(c) 7. *I odnose i prenose,*
     8. *Preko mora bez odmora —*

(d) 9. *Gde macka ne mauce,*
    10. *Gde svinjce ne gurice,*
    11. *Gde ovce ne bleje,*
    12. *Gde koze ne vrece,*

(e) 13. *Gde pop ne dolazi,*
    14. *Gde krst ne donosi,*
    15. *Da se kolac ne lomi,*
    16. *Da se svece ne pali.*

(f) 17. *Bezi boljku u polje,*
    18. *Bezi boljku u more,*
    19. *Bezi boljku pod kamen;*
    20. *Tu ti mesta nema!*

(g) 21. *Otud ide crvena krava,*
    22. *Crveno tele otelila,*
    23. *Crveno mleko podojila.*

(h) 24. *Otud ide crvena kvocka,*
    25. *Vode devet crvenih pilica,*
    26. *Padose na crveni bunjak,*
    27. *Pokupise crveni crvici.*

(c) 28. *I odnese preko mora,*
    29. *Preko mora bez odmora.*

(f) 30. *(Idi) Bezi vetra u polje,*
    31. *Bezi vetra u more,*
    32. *Bezi vetra;*
    33. *Tu ti mesta nema!*

(i) — *[(ime) ostaje]*
    34. *Lako kao pero,*
    35. *Cisti kao srebro,*
    36. *Blazi kao materno mleko.*

(j) 37. *Otud ide Ugimir,*
    38. *Ugini boljku, ugini!*
    39. *Otud ide Stanimir,*
    40. *Stani boljku, stani!*
    41. *Otud ide Persa,*
    42. *Prestani boljku, prestani!*

(k) 43. *Deset, devet, osam, sedam,*
    44. *Sest, pet, cet'ri, tri, dva, jedan.*

(l) 45. *U kurjaka cet'ri noge, peti rep,*
    46. *Od mog odgovora bio lek!*

NOTES AND REFERENCES

1 See, for example, C. M. Bowra, *Primitive Song*, Cleveland, World, 1962; and O. Cockayne, *Leechdoms, Wortcunning, and Starcraft of Early England*, Vol. I., Wiesbaden, Klaus (reprint from 1864 London ed.), 1965.

2 Research has been carried out under National Endowment for the Humanities grant no. RC-20505-74-552. Field work took place under the aegis of participation by Joel M. Halpern in an exchange programme between the National Academy of Sciences, Washington, D.C., and the Serbian Academy of Sciences, Belgrade, during summer 1975. We acknowledge with particular appreciation the co-operation of the host academy in endorsement of the field phase of the project.

3 See J. M. Pavlovic, *Zivot i obicaji narodni u Kragujevackoj Jasenici u Sumadiji*, Belgrade, Srpska Kraljevska Akademija, 1921; P. Kemp, *Healing Ritual: Studies in the Technique and Tradition of the Southern Slavs*, London, Faber & Faber, 1935; A. Petrovic, *Rakovica: socijalno-zdravstvene i higijenske prilike*, Belgrade, Biblioteka Centralnog Higijenskog Zavoda, 1939; P. Z. Petrovic, *Zivot i obicaji narodni u Gruzi*, Belgrade, Srpska Akademija Nauka, 1948; and S. Knezevic and M. Jovanovic, *Jarmenovci*, Belgrade, Srpska Akademija Nauka, 1958.

4 Of the Serbo-Croation oral epic Albert Lord (*The Singer of Tales*, New York, Atheneum, 1968) remarks: 'The song we are listening to is "the song"; for each performance is more than a performance; it is a re-creation. . . . Both synchronically and historically there would be numerous creations and re-creations of the song. This concept of the relationship between "songs" (performances of the same specific or generic song) is closer to the truth than the concept of an "original" and "variants". In a sense, each performance is "an" original, if not "the" original' (p. 101).

In a similar vein, we have selected what seems to us to be the most characteristic version among eight variants of the particular charm elicited. The text of the performance presented here in English translation (and in the original Serbo-Croatian in an Appendix) is, therefore, 'the charm' for our purposes.

For examples of related performances of a range of songs by the same and different epic singers collected at various times, see also M. Parry and A. B. Lord (trans. and ed.), *Serbo-Croatian Heroic Songs* (*Srpskohrvatske junacke pesme*), Vols. I & II, Cambridge and Belgrade, Harvard University Press and Serbian Academy of Sciences, 1954.

5 J. M. Halpern and B. K. Halpern, *A Serbian Village in Historical Perspective*, New York, Holt, Rinehart & Winston, 1972; see also J. M. Foley and B. K. Halpern, '*Udovica Jana*: a case study of an oral performance', *Slavonic and East European Review*, Vol. 54, 1976, pp. 11-23.

6 See Appendix, p. 00.

7 See C. Lévi-Strauss, 'The effectiveness of symbols', in *Structural Anthropology*, New York, Anchor Books, 1967, pp. 181-201.

8   Note that the Serbo-Croatian *lek* (medicine) is cognate with early modern English leech, which in turn derives from Old English *læcdom*, the practice of curing. Under the latter designation were included healing charms very similar in structure and function to the charm presented here.

9   See, for example, J. Obrebski, *Field notes on research in a Macedonian village* (unpublished), Amherst, Archives of University of Massachusetts Library, 1932-33, and Kemp, op. cit.

10   A survey of brides' villages of origin shows that about two-thirds of rural brides marry outside their natal villages and within a radius of 20-25 miles. J. M. Halpern and B. K. Halpern, *A Serbian Village,* New York, Harper & Row, 1967.

11   For similar attitudes in rural Greece see Richard Blum and Eva Blum, *The Dangerous Hour: the Lore and Culture of Crisis and Mystery in Rural Greece,* New York, Scribner, 1970, p. 351. Compare Obrebski, who observed in a Macedonian village: '. . . to be fully effective the spells must be transmitted in the performer's mother's line, "from my faith and from my blood".' J. Obrebski, 'Social structure and ritual in a Macedonian village', trans. and ed. by B. K. Halpern, posthumous paper given at 1969 meeting of American Association for the Advancement of Slavic Studies, Boston, p. 15.

12   Often in the course of field work we reassured informants that the tapes were being recorded for our use only, that we were interested in the charms as examples of traditional poetry and as part of history. 'Well, if that's the way it is,' one woman agreed. 'But you know what it's like here in the village – if that black Radojka were to find out that I know this charm, she'd be jealous, and who knows what evil spell she'd work on me!'

13   See, for example, M. Douglas, *Purity and Danger,* London, Routledge & Kegan Paul, 1966; and V. W. Turner, *The Drums of Affliction,* Oxford, Clarendon Press, 1968.

14   See also A. Petrovic, op. cit., p. 79.

15   It is interesting to note that Marko has absorbed the charm structure simply by having been present on many occasions when Desanka performed the healing ritual. As a male, he would not have been formally taught the basma, and will never practise *bajanje* in the future. This ability to internalize traditional genres, even when age and sex roles preclude active performance of the material, is characteristic of the members of an oral culture (see also J. M. Foley, 'The traditional oral audience', *Balkan Studies,* Vol. 17, forthcoming).

16   All versions of the charm reveal a composite structure of a series of internally coherent and externally related motifs, which we enumerate as follows:

(a) *horse and rider*
(b) *as/so*
(c) *carry*
(d) *animal catalogue*
(e) *Christian catalogue*

(f) *banishment*
(g) *cow motif*
(h) *hen motif*
(i) *purification*
(j) *symbolic names*
(k) *inverted counting*
(l) *wolf*

These motifs or frames tend towards prosodic units of four octosyllabic lines each and demonstrate relatively uniform actualization from one version to the next. Variations depend upon the identiy of the frame, the immediate textual environment, and the performance situation.

17   For the Serbo-Croatian original see Appendix. A thorough contrastive linguistic analysis of two versions of this charm, along with detailed examination of process in oral transmission as demonstrated by six additional versions by the same performer over an eight-day period, will appear in our forthcoming article 'Power of the Word: Healing Charms as an Oral Genre'.

18   Kemp, op. cit., p. 36.

19   M. Eliade, *The Sacred and the Profane: the Nature of Religion,* trans. by W. R. Trask, New York, Harcourt, Brace & World, 1959.

20   Trans. from V. S. Karadzic, *Zivot i obicaji naroda Srpskoga,* Belgrade, Srpska Knjizevna Zadruga, 1957, p. 233. On this very common mythic motif, often termed the 'night sea journey', see C. G. Jung, *Symbols of Transformation,* trans. by R. F. C. Hull, *The Collected Works of C. G. Jung,* Vol. 5, Princeton, Princeton University Press, 1967, pp. 210 ff., and the original exposition by L. Frobenius, *Das Zeitalter des Sonnengottes,* Vol. 1, Berlin, 1904, pp. 30 ff.

21   Conjurers indentify ritual times of day for the practice of *bajanje;* our field work indicates that the designated time varies (both among *bajalice* and among diseases). Most common, however, is *po podne* ('after noon'), when the sun begins its downward motion.

22   In S. Kulisic, P. Z. Petrovic and N. Pantelic, *Srpski mitoloski recnik,* Belgrade, Nolit, 1970, p. 82.

23   Ibid.; Kemp, op. cit., p. 143.

24   This text as presented is faithful to the form in which it was transmitted orally and received aurally. As such, it contains several phonological and syntactic deviations from standard Serbo-Croatian. The motivation for these and other 'mistakes' in transmission is discussed by the authors in another article; see note 17.

Donn V. Hart

4

Disease Etiologies of Samaran Filipino Peasants [1]

Introduction

The main purpose of this chapter is to examine the folk explanations for the causes of disease or illness (*sakit* or *mara-ot eton lawas*) that are accepted by the residents of a Filipino village in Eastern Samar Island. The analysis is in light of George Foster's proposal that non-Western disease etiologies are characterized by either *personalistic* or *naturalistic* principles.

A secondary purpose, essential to achieving the first, is to present a comprehensive, if abbreviated, outline of ethnomedicine in this peasant community. This summary includes not only the etiologies of most locally recognized diseases, but also their diagnosis, varied treatment and associated curers. The data for this chapter were gathered in this village in 1955-56 and partly updated in 1977. [2]

The Setting

The central islands of the Philippine archipelago (e.g. Panay, Negros, Cebu, Bohol, Leyte and Samar) are known collectively as the Bisayas and their inhabitants as Bisayans. Within the Bisayas, Samar and eastern Leyte are settled by a cultural-linguistic group called Samarans. [3] Samar, whose eastern coast faces the open Pacific Ocean, is the third largest island in the Philippines. Eastern Samar province, our research area, is a series of small deltaic lowlands, partially divided by mountain spurs stretching from the

57

densely forested central highland to the Pacific. Lalawigan is a village (*barrio*) of 889 persons in 187 households (author's census, 1956). It is located five miles south of Eastern Samar's provincial capital, Borongan.

Lalawigan's economy is based on the production of *copra* (dried coconut meat), *abaca* (Manila hemp), and rice. In-shore non-motorized fishing is another major economic activity. Most residences are of bamboo and palm thatch raised above the ground on sturdy poles. Kinship is traced bilaterally and the nuclear family is the most important social unit. No type of unilineal organization exists. All Lalawignons are Roman Catholics. In 1956 the nearest priest resided in Borongan. Each house has a family altar with saint figures and pictures of the Holy Family. The altar is the focus of household religious activities. Social life mainly involves the various life crises (baptisms, marriages, funerals, etc.), the annual fiesta for the patron saint of the community, the Catholic religious calendar and public school functions.

Causes of Illness

In a personalistic medical system, according to Foster, sickness is explained as resulting from the

> *active, purposeful intervention* of an *agent,* who may be human (a witch or sorcerer), nonhuman (a ghost, an ancestor, an evil spirit), or supernatural (a deity or other very powerful being). The sick person literally is a victim, the object of aggression or punishment directed specifically against him, for reasons that concern him alone. Personalistic causality allows little room for accident or chance. . . .[4]

The etiological system of Lalawigan, in this aspect, is primarily personalistic. Although detailed statistics on morbidity were not collected in Lalawigan, extensive interviews, household census data, and participant observation indicated that the causes of the majority of serious illnesses were believed to be actions of environmental spirits, sorcerers (and their familiars or 'pets'), and ancestral souls. Sickness was diagnosed, either by the patient, a family member, or the curers, as punishment for offences against these various agents. A description of these agents, and their disease-creating powers, is now provided.

Environmental Spirits

Maglimbunganon (from *maglimbung*, a cheat or deceiver) is the generic name in Lalawigan for the environmental spirits who inhabit the land (trees, caves, rivers, springs, etc.) and the sea. These spirits are usually referred to in everyday conversation (often to avoid using their real names) as 'People who are not like us' or *mara-ot nga tawo* (bad persons). The invisible spirits (that may and do show themselves at will) resemble tall humans, often Spanish or American *mestizos* (i.e. Filipinos one of whose direct ancestors, usually the father, was a Spaniard or an American). With the exception of their supernatural powers, the spirits' lifestyle is almost identical to that of mortal Filipinos. Some are farmers, others fishermen; they marry, have children, christen their young as Catholics, gamble at the cockpit, grow old and die. They dress like Filipinos and eat the same diet except that their food is never salted. Some spirits are poor, although others (probably the majority) live in spacious, elaborately furnished mansions. They drive automobiles and fly airplanes. Although the origin of these spirits is pre-Hispanic (and pan-Southeast Asian), the barriofolk through reinterpretation have made them members of the folk Catholic pantheon of supernatural beings.[5]

Environmental spirits in eastern Samar are also commonly named after their primary residence (see Table 1). *Dagatnon* or *lawodon* who live in the sea rarely cause sickness, perhaps because their contacts with humans are limited. They are believed to be the 'masters' of the fish; fishermen have various rituals relating to the *dagatnon* to ensure successful fishing activities.[6] One variety of *tunanon*, the *botbot*, is similar to 'a giant worm' that makes the earth tremble when it moves. Its name is derived from the sound it makes when moving – '*bot-bot-bot*'. During late afternoon or at twilight, the *botbot's* head or nose may protrude above ground. If one accidentally steps on the *botbot*, a boil or abcess occurs.

TABLE 1

Varieties of Environmental Spirits in Lalawigan

Names	Residences
Dagatnon, lawodnon	*Dagat,* sea water, or *lawod,* sea or a large body of water
Tunan-on	*Tuna,* earth
Kahoynon	*Kahoy,* tree
Guban-on	*Guba,* forest
Lungibnon	*Lungib,* cave

Kahoynon usually live only in large trees such as the balete, *lauan, dungon,* and *da-o.* The most virulent of all *kahoynon* is the *tugopnon* that resides in the *tugop* tree. This spirit is unusually ugly, has a twisted nose, a fair skin covered with red or black spots, and wears a G-string. There are also three types of *kahoynon* known as *dalakitnon* (*dalakit,* balete tree, *Ficus payapa* Blanco). [7]

Although the *guban-on* live in the forest, they rarely inhabit trees. One variety of *guban-on,* called *tahoy* (*pagtaghoy,* to whistle), is reputedly a tall, thin spirit with a 'sharp face like a bird'. One type of *lungibnon* is the *agta,* a fierce, tall, black-skinned savage who wears a necklace of centipedes and clothing of bark. *Agta* are hirsute with silky head hair touching their shoulders. On the whole, they do not hurt humans but delight in frightening or playing pranks on the barriofolk, for example, making one lose one's way. [8]

Usually, these spirits are described as 'evil' in the Philippine literature, although many are neutral towards humans until molested, offended or disturbed. The intent of one's action towards them is irrevelant. 'A traveler in the forest who innocently and injudiciously urinates on their [invisible] gardens is struck down as ruthlessly as a person who consciously violates their domain.' [9]

Although these spirits rarely sicken humans unless provoked, they live everywhere around them (although not within the barrio), so often it is difficult not to offend them. To live Lalawignons must fish, open new swiddens in the mountains, cut bamboo, travel in the forest, etc. Since the spirits and their residences are invisible, one must constantly be alert not to antagonize them, invade their privacy, or destroy their property. A wise person avoids, whenever possible, known spirit habitation sites, e.g. certain trees, springs, or caves.[10] It is best not to work during the afternoon siesta since the spirits are peeved if their naps are disturbed. If possible, one should not wander outside the house or around the barrio at night, for this is when spirits (and sorcerers) are most active. However, during a lifetime, no matter how careful one may be, it is impossible not to enrage some of these vengeful spirits.

No one ailment is attributed to any specific category of spirits. On the other hand, if one were in the forest, cutting bamboo or planting a swidden, and shortly thereafter became ill, the suspected agent would be a *kahoynon* or *guban-on*. Many etiologies, for this reason, are based on situational or behavioural factors preceding the sickness. In Lalawigan, as in eastern Negros Island,[11] known or putative contacts with the spirits are usually more important in diagnosis than symptoms of the ailment. Some illnesses, however, are invariably attributed to the spirits, e.g. the intrusion of invisible foreign objects. known as *turok* or *hangin,* into the patient's body. Another ailment is believed to be caused only by the spirits. When a human is befriended by a spirit (known as *sinasangkayan*) mental illness occurs. (Incidentally this is an exception to the rule that the spirits never harm a human unless offended.)

Souls (*Kalag*)

Other illnesses in Lalawigan are traced to the punitive action of angered and vengeful ancestral souls: 'Souls may punish their descendants since they can talk with God.' Briefly, souls cause sickness primarily for violation of generally accepted values, e.g. disrespect of one's elders, failing to care for sickly or aged parents, dishonesty, physical violence (stabbings, etc.), incestuous marriages (such as first cousins), or failure to hold proper rituals. Rituals for the souls are regarded, in part, as 'rent' paid them for the inherited land presently farmed by their descendants. Souls that are properly respected by the living in deed and action and are honoured by these rituals reward their descendants with abundant harvests, healthy and multiplying children and farm animals (chickens, pigs, carabao, etc.) and general good fortune.

According to the barriofolk the rituals for these souls (usually a novena, i.e. nine consecutive evenings of prayer or a rosary) have two purposes. One is to remember the anniversaries of the deaths of all of one's ancestors; the other is to maintain a close, intimate relationship among living kinsmen. In pursuit of these two purposes the *katig-uban* (*tig-ub*, to add), once popular but rarely held today, used to be organized by several families in memory of their deceased relatives. It was said that in the past, when Lalawigan was less populous, one *katig-uban* was held for the souls of all the deceased residents of the village. Today the more common ritual is the *katu-igan* (*tuig*, year, or 'yearly') held by a single family for its souls. Sometimes a *katu-igan* is started on the recommendation of the shaman when the cause of a family member's sickness is diagnosed as angered ancestral souls. In some instances the sickness may be traced to a particular soul. For example, the 'orphan soul' (*ilo nga kalag*) of a childless man or woman may sicken a sibling for neglect to perform rituals.

Once a *katu-igan* is done it must be repeated annually. The duty is 'inherited' along with the other property one receives from a deceased person. All members of the family should attend the *katu-igan*. If return to Lalawigan is impossible, absent members may light a candle in a church in their community and recite a prayer for the souls. Some Lalawignons working in Manila return for the annual *katu-igan,* especially if they have been 'sickly' or have had 'sleepless nights'. In the past an elaborate food offering was part of the *katig-uban.*[12] Only a snack is served at the *katu-igan.*[13]

A blameless person may become ill through the action of a specific ancestral soul despite an affectionate past relationship. For example, a dead mother who was inordinately fond of one of her children, perhaps the 'pet', or a deceased grandparent who cared for and was unusually devoted to a grandchild, may 'long' for the child to join them. In this instance sickness is not the result of an offence but of loving souls' desire to be reunited with loved ones. For example, one sick young man in Lalawigan claimed he saw an old woman lying next to his sleeping mat. The more he gazed upon this figure, invisible to all but him, the sicker he became. The shaman decided that the ghostly figure was his maternal grandmother who 'longed' for her grandson whom she had reared. After the parents held a novena for their maternal grandparents, their son recovered. It is also said that living kinsmen, separated from a loved one, may 'long' for a reunion so intensely that they sicken the desired person.

The preceding section has summarized disease etiologies traced either to non-human entities such as environmental spirits or to ancestral souls. However, many sicknesses are blamed on humans with preternatural powers, particularly on the sorcerers known as *barangan* and *sigbinan*. Their roles in the traditional etiological system of Lalawigan are now discussed.

Sorcerers: Barangan

Sorcerers known as *barangan* and *sigbinan* are blamed for numerous illnesses occurring in Lalawigan. The *barangan* is discussed first.[14]

This sorcerer (always a male) may on his own account sicken (sometimes to death) humans he dislikes. More typically his powers are used against the victim at the request of others. *Barangan* can be hired to retaliate against those who have attacked or slandered a client or his close kinsmen, stolen their property, etc.

The *barangan* purchases his vicious 'pets', insects called *tawa* (similar to the rice weevil, *bokbok*), that are kept in a bottle of coconut oil. When the *barangan* wishes his insects to attack a victim, he inserts a small wooden cross in the neck of the bottle. He then instructs his 'pets': 'You are my servants and I have someone to punish.' He gives the name (and describes the physical features) of the victim and tells the insects where the victim lives. The insects are then sent on their gory errand. If they return to the *barangan* covered with blood, it means they successfully penetrated the victim's body. The *barangan* also has the power to 'shoot' invisible foreign objects into the victim's body. Typical ailments associated with *binarang* (the act of being sorcerized by the *barangan*) are sores, body swelling, and painful joints, and especially diseases that result in leprosy-like disfigurements of the face.[15]

The *barangan,* as is typical of others with supernatural powers, is subject to a number of constraints. He cannot enter a church for ten years after the purchase of his 'pets'. During this period he cannot eat salted food and must fast on certain days. After the first

decade, the sorcerer may attend church services but he must leave
before Christ is consecrated during the mass. He never permits
anyone to secure any of his loose hair and expectorates into a bottle.
Hair, saliva, and other personal items may be used by a sorcerer to
cast a spell on an individual.

Sickness caused by the intrusion of foreign objects into the
victim's body, through the actions of environmental spirits or the
barangan, is called *hangin, turok,* or *to-onay.* Its treatment is
known as *haplas.* An angered spirit, using a 'bad' wind (*hangin*)
also 'shoots' (*turok,* pierce) or 'sows' dirt (*dahora*) in the victim's
body. The objects enter the body without making a wound; when
they are extracted no bleeding occurs. The patient may diagnose
his own illness, consult the shaman, or seek treatment from a
specialist in this disease (the *haplasan* or *parahaplas*). One patient
claimed he had forty thorns removed from his body. Another informant had a large sore on his foot. After treatment a centipede
emerged from the lesion. *Haplas* is also used to treat certain skin
diseases.

Symptoms of *hangin* or *turok* are an initial cold, with fever and
headaches, followed by aches and pains in the muscles and joints.
There are four methods to treat this sickness. First and second, the
healer removes the objects with a needle ('the most painful way') or
his fingers; third, medicinal coconut oil (sometimes called *lana nga
eharaplas*)[16] and 'smoking' are used; and fourth, herbal medicines
are used, either as a poultice or as a liquid that is drunk. There are
also home remedies for *hangin,* particularly if the initial affliction
is not serious. For example, one woman explained that she removed thorns from under an eye by applying half of a cut citrus-
like fruit, *makalpi* (similar to *kahil*). Another similar remedy is to
heat *paleyo* leaves (from a small shrub whose cut branches 'quickly
wilt' if not put in water) and apply them to the sore spot.

One *parahaplas* in Lalawigan removed foreign objects from
her patients' bodies with her finger. (The prefix *para* means 'one
who does'.) After the objects were extracted, she 'smoked' the
patient with *ambal* (ambergris?). Sometimes Tiger Balm (a popular Asian ointment) is also massaged on the sore spots. She
required her patients to remain in her residence for three days after
the treatment. Space permits only a partial listing of the various
herbal concoctions used to treat *hangin.*[17]

When medicinal coconut oil is to be used to treat *hangin,* the patient first bathes and then dresses in clean clothes. The patient then either lies on a white sheet or the afflicted spots are covered with white cloths after a massage with coconut oil. Sometimes the curer makes the sign of the cross with coconut oil on the patient's tongue. While under the sheet the patient may also be 'smoked', as in the treatment of *lanti*. Later the foreign objects appear on the sheet or cloths. This treatment should be repeated for three consecutive days; each session takes about an hour. (One informant reported, however, that he was treated for *hangin* three times in one day – 'I was in a hurry to get well for the fiesta was coming.') The extracted objects are burned, for they can infect others. Informants claim that once one is treated with *haplas,* the treatment 'becomes a habit'. It must be repeated in the future, without any choice on the part of the patient if the illness is diagnosed as *hangin* or *turok.*

Sigbinan

The second kind of human agent responsible for illness (and death) is the *sigbinan*.[18] They are men or women who inherit from their parents small, fantastic, puppy-like creatures covered with fine hair whose bite is venomous — 'far more poisonous than a centipede bite'. These creatures often are called 'puppies' when the *sigbinan* are discussed. Many families in the barrio who had lost children in their infancy attributed one or more of these deaths to *sigbin* bites. One mother claimed that three of her children had died in this way, while in another family four children had died from *sigbin* bites. Although *sigbins* may bite adults (especially if children are not available), they rarely die from the venom. The *sigbinan* are said to prefer infants or small children since they cannot explain what causes their illness and 'are more susceptible to the poison'.[19]

    Sigbins are dangerous in Lalawigan because their owners are too poor or too lazy to feed them, so the creatures are forced to seek human victims. Rarely, if ever, does the *sigbinan* use his animals to punish people who have offended him; he cannot be hired by others as may a *barangan*. During the day their owners keep the *sigbins* in a large earthenware jar (*tadyao*). When the *sigbins* are fed, they are given chicken or carabao meat at midnight. *Sigbins* eat only during the periods of the new and full moon. It is at this time that the *sigbinan* may put his 'pets' in a basket and go in search of possible victims. The *sigbinan* substitutes a banana stalk or another object that looks exactly like the victim's corpse. The corpse is taken by the *sigbinan* to feed his animals. Since the *sigbinan* shares the corpse with the *sigbins,* they are considered cannibals and have a 'pale appearance'.

In 1977 some Lalawignons claimed a man was seen walking along the beach in the early morning, carrying a basket on his back. From the basket dangled two small hands that moved. Behind the *sigbinan* followed his 'pets' which kept biting the exposed hands of the child that was still alive. Informants claimed that the *sigbinan* was taking the child home so that the *sigbins* and he could feast on it.

The *sigbinan* can become invisible, 'hide under a stick' or 'pass through a hole as small as the one in a needle'. They are able to travel rapidly; it is difficult to catch a *sigbinan* since his body is slippery from the coconut oil (*lana*) he applies before leaving home. A *sigbinan* cannot die until one of his children agrees to inherit his animals 'just like they do any other property'. If the *sigbin* are buried with their owner, they later return home. They cannot be drowned or burned; such attempts only result in their multiplication.

The *sigbin* may bite its victim in any part of the body, but the favourite spots are the nape of the neck, below the ear, or on the cheek. Bites are more virulent in these areas than elsewhere on the body. The symptoms of a *sigbin* bite are a high fever, spasms, difficulty in breathing ('one feels pressed'), etc. The bitten area does not throb or swell as is typical of a centipede or spider bite. Some parents move a child bitten by a *sigbin* to a relative's house because the *sigbin* will return if the victim does not die. Unless the bite can be located, the victim dies, since herbal medicines are ineffective unless applied directly to the wound. Frequently the bites are invisible, appearing only after the patient has died. However, one shaman claimed he could locate an invisible bite 'because heat is concentrated in that spot'.

Once the patient's ailment is diagnosed as a *sigbin* bite, various treatments are possible. Although this illness is common in the barrio, no traditional curer specialized solely in its treatment. Some parents treat their children, but most request the diagnostic and therapeutic services of *sunahan,* a curer specializing in treating all poisonous bites. Medicine purchased in Borongan for poisonous snake and insect bites may be used, including Vicks. Other patent medicines are bought from travelling Boholan peddlars who visit the barrio.

Various herbal concoctions are used to treat *sigbin* bites. The leaves, bark, new shoots, and roots of numerous plants are soaked in water (hot or cold) or in blessed vinegar.[20] The water or vinegar is either administered orally or rubbed on the bite area. Sometimes heated leaves (or their juice) are applied to the bite.[21] 'Smoking' (*paglo-on*) is another treatment for a *sigbin* bite. Certain herbs are put in a coconut shell with live coals. The patient is then 'bathed' or 'smoked' with the fumes. A hair from the *sigbin* (if available), a pungent sap (*ingo-ingo*), or a feather of a supposedly poisonous bird (*obonobon*) may be added to the coals. As much as possible the fumes should be directed to the bitten area of the body. One mother advised that in treating the patient, only the third finger (three is a magical number in the barrio) should be used to rub the body.[22] During this treatment the sign of the cross may be traced on various parts of the patient's body.

If the *sigbin* bite is visible, treatment normally results in a cure. One additional complication of *sigbin* bites is that the child may become apprehensive and develop *lanti,* an emotional disturbance caused by fright.

It is impossible to classify disease etiologies in Lalawigan as of wholly pre- or wholly post-Hispanic origin. The environmental spirits are certainly pre-Hispanic (and pan-Southeast Asian), yet the barriofolk have reinterpreted their origin on the basis of their folk Catholicism. Therapy for illnesses caused by the spirits includes many post-Hispanic, especially Catholic, elements. Pre-Hispanic Filipinos were equally solicitous in maintaining amicable relationships with ancestral souls, although today these are placated primarily by Catholic rites. However, the etiologies of some illnesses of a personalistic character appear post-Hispanic, the result of the Christianization of the Filipinos. These sources of sickness are briefly described next.

Sins Against God

The role of God as a disease agent appears to vary among different Christian Filipino groups. Jocano claims that *'Diyos,* or God, is often seen as a revengeful environmental spirit' who causes illness.[23] This belief was found in a story in a Philippine elementary school reader.[24] Lieban mentions that only a 'few illnesses' are attributed to God.[25] A psychologist writes that the notion of sin does not seem 'especially salient in the Philippines and a disease theory based on such a concept might not be a very powerful one'.[26] Finally, Nurge found in her east Leyte community that 'No ailment was ever reported to be a visitation from God as a punishment for sin or as a trial of one's faith, ideas prominent in some Christian circles.'[27]

In Lalawigan the barriofolk believe all sickness can be traced indirectly to God. In fact, everything that happens to one is the result of God's will. Yet God is rarely (if ever) petitioned to punish an individual with sickness. However, a person may pray to St Antonio, San Roque, Mary or the patron saint of Borongan to punish another with sickness. Lalawignons pray to St Antonio to cure the sick; the assumption is that since St Antonio can cure, he also can sicken. One holds a novena for the saint. During the prayers the image is stuck with a pin in the part of the body where one wishes the victim to suffer. No specific sickness is associated with these saints and such petitions are rare, made only when one has been gravely offended. Some informants claim that this method is used only to punish thieves. Two women in Lalawigan were claimed to be skilled in this technique. In fact, one allegedly caused a cousin, who had stolen her *copra,* to have a mental disorder. In 1977 a person who had been ill for nearly a year consulted several *tambalans* who told him his malady was the result of prayers to a saint. The patient was advised to go to the person he had offended to request forgiveness for his sin.

Gaba

Gaba, another cause of illness and general misfortune in Lalawigan, is mainly limited to younger couples. *Gaba* is initiated by an offended person who petitions God to punish one who has wronged him with illness.[28] The major causes of *gaba* (more common among kinsmen than non-kinsmen) are when a younger person is disrespectful towards an elderly person, especially his parents, towards those born with physical defects, or when he wastes food. For example, *gaba* may sicken a child who quarrels with or disobeys his parents, steals, marries without parental permission, ridicules a cripple, etc.[29] In some cases the offending person may escape punishment but it will be afflicted on his children. If one suspects illness is due to *gaba* (no specific ailment is associated solely with *gaba*), the cure is to request forgiveness from the offended person. For example, if a woman suspects *gaba* is the reason for a difficult pregnancy, the wronged person is requested, after forgiveness is granted, to touch her swollen abdomen with a finger.

Gaba is not a frequent cause of illness in Lalawigan. However, one woman used *gaba* to punish her daughter's husband's brother for stealing from her. His body swelled and he died in a few days. In retaliation the deceased man's wife invoked *gaba* against this woman, resulting in the death of two (some say three) of her children.

Finally, *gaba* may cause misfortune, not sickness. One who wastes food may be punished with meagre harvests or consistently bad luck in fishing.

The preceding sections of this chapter have summarized numerous personalistic etiologies. Our research did not systematically collect detailed statistics on the frequencies of various illnesses (or on the causes of death) in this village. However, a conservative estimate (based on observation, interviews with both informants and curers, and household censuses) is that the barriofolk explained about 65 per cent of all serious ailments (and deaths) in this village as the result of actions by supernatural entities of sorcerers. The two most common agents probably are the environmental spirits and *sigbinan*.

Lalawigan data also confirm Foster's proposition that 'in personalistic systems *illness is but a special case in the explanation of all misfortune*'.[30] The spirits and ancestral souls have the power both to reward and punish humans. In most instances the spirits punish only when Filipinos violate their domain or anger them.

When they and their invisible world are avoided or respected, the spirits can and do reward the barriofolk. Numerous examples of the beneficial actions of spirits were reported. For example, the healing powers of some shaman are gifts of friendly spirits (and souls). A bountiful swidden harvest cannot be achieved without the co-operation of the *kahoynons*. One resident allegedly had a spirit as his compadre; as a result he was quite prosperous. One sympathetic spirit thoughtfully left a meal for a group of hungry harvesters. A fisherman with a *katao*[31] as a friend always has full traps and nets: 'We all use the same equipment and fishing technique yet these two brothers *always* have bigger catches.'

Finally, the environmental spirits do not inflict sickness on Lalawignons for social deviancy. A thief, murderer or adulterer would not be punished by the spirits with illness for his misdeeds. When illness is diagnosed as a result of such wrongdoing, the agents identified are ancestral souls, saints, or sorcerers. For those who follow faithfully the 'old customs', the souls are a source of support and benefit. All one must do, to avoid sickness or other forms of misfortune by these agents, is to honour the basic values they cherished when among the living. In many societies illness is conceived as punishment for violating accepted values.[32] The Filipino social order is also identified with the moral order of the universe; health is the reward for conformity.[33]

Foster wisely recognized that '*the two etiologies* [personalistic and naturalistic] *are rarely if ever mutually exclusive* as far as their presence or absence in a particular society is concerned. People who invoke personalistic causes to explain most illness usually recognize some natural, or chance, causes.'[34] He distinguishes between the two systems.

> In contrast to personalistic systems, naturalistic systems explain illness in impersonal, systemic terms. Disease is thought to stem, not from the machinations of an angry being, but rather from such *natural forces or conditions* as cold, heat, winds, dampness, and, above all, from an upset in the balance of the basic body elements.[35]

He continues by stating that 'In naturalistic systems, health conforms to an *equilibrium* model: ... Causality concepts explain or account for the upsets in this balance that trigger illness.'[36] One illustrative example he suggests is humoral pathology. Since in an earlier monograph I reported in detail on humoral pathology as part of the traditional etiological system of Lalawigan and elsewhere in the Philippines, this chapter gives only a brief summary of this 'Great Tradition' medical complex.[37]

Humoral Pathology

Greek humoral pathology was brought to Spain by its Muslim conquerors (eighth to eleventh centuries); from there it diffused to Latin America during the Conquest (sixteenth to seventeeth centuries). For the most part, humoral pathology concepts in the Philippines were carried from Latin America (or directly from Spain) after most of the archipelago was conquered by the Spaniards in the sixteenth century.[38]

Lalawignons believe that good health requires the proper balance between 'hot' and 'cold' elements in the body. If this balance is disturbed, illness occurs. Numerous rules exist on how to retain a 'healthy' balance of these elements in the body. For example, various foods and diseases are classified as 'hot', 'cold', or 'neutral or regular'. Some 'hot' foods are chicken, duck and squash (*ampalaya*); 'cold' foods include beef, goat, cucumbers and eggplant; and some 'regular' foods are cabbage and rice.[39] Beri-beri and stomach-ache are 'cold' illnesses; fever, malaria, and tuberculosis are 'hot' ones; boils, flu (colds), and earaches may be either 'hot' or 'cold'. Only 'cold' foods or medicines should be taken to counteract a 'hot' disease.

Even the most fastidious observation of this metaphysical 'equilibrium' does not assure good health since many etiologies, as already described, are personalistic. Some diseases have multiple etiologies. For example, dysentery may be caused by overeating (especially of fruit) during the summer when food is abundant, by 'thorn' projectiles 'shot' into the body by the spirits or *barangan,* or by excessive 'heat' in the body, often blamed on failure to take a daily bath (see Table 2). Finally, the barriofolk do not use humoral pathology to explain misfortunes other than illness.[40]

The dichotomy of etiologies as either personalistic or naturalistic is not always clear-cut.

Most troublesome, at least at first glance, are those illnesses believed caused by emotional disturbances such as fright, jealousy, envy, shame, anger, or grief. Fright, or *susto,* widespread in Latin America, can be caused by a ghost, a spirit, or an encounter with the devil; if the agent *intended* harm to the victim, the etiology is certainly personalistic. But often accounts of such encounters suggest chance or accident rather than purposive action.[41]

Again, Lalawigan offers an excellent example of a sickness based on emotional upsts.

Lanti is a common illness allegedly caused by fright (*hadlok*).[42] With a few exceptions, this ailment sickens only infants or young children. The illness is not fatal in itself, but if the patient is not cured he may weaken physically until he succumbs from another cause. The etiology of *lanti* is not traced to the environmental spirits, ancestral souls, or humans with supernatural powers. There are two causes of *lanti.* First, the child is directly frightened, e.g. by seeing two men fight, barking dogs, a large fire with black clouds of smoke, falling into a ditch, tumbling out of a bamboo 'walker', or hearing a sudden loud noise. *Lanti* is also caused indirectly when a permanent member of the child's household is frightened. Some typical examples that have resulted in the transference of fright to the child are when a household member saw or killed a large snake, was attacked by an infuriated carabao, helped put a body of a neighbour into his coffin, visited a large cave, or fired a gun.

Most Lalawignons are uncertain why *lanti* is restricted to the youngest child or how someone else's fright is transferred to him. One informant speculated that the transference was a process 'like magnetism'. Most barriofolk think the diffusion of fright occurs because the involved individuals are kinsmen, live permanently in the same household, and have an intimate relationship with the child. The principle of contagious magic best explains this invisible bond that channels fright from one member of the household to the youngest child.

In other societies this magic affinity is regarded as existing among related persons, among agemates, and among members of social groups of many other kinds. Whatever good or harm befalls objects or individuals of one class also befalls other members of the class without any necessary direct contact, unless magical preventive measures are taken.[43]

Lanti has many symptoms but curers who specialize in treating it claim that the three most recurrent symptoms are fever, boils, and reddish blotches where the skin folds on the arms, legs, and neck. When a child is ill either the parents or a curer diagnoses the sickness. The treatments are too esoteric to be handled by home remedies. The three kinds of Lalawigan specialists in *lanti* and how they treat this sickness have been described elsewhere.[44] The practitioners who treat only *lanti* have no supernatural source of their knowledge and skills. The curing rites are neither the gift of a spirit nor learned from a sorcerer. It is obvious *lanti* should be classified as having a naturalistic etiology.

Disease and Supernaturalism

Literature on folk medicine, including most sources for the Philippines, usually emphasizes that it is impossible to separate into discrete categories beliefs and practices associated with disease and supernaturalism (magic and religion). The presence of intricate linkages between supernaturalism and disease is a diagnostic trait of personalistic medical systems.[45] In comparison, naturalistic medical systems make little use of supernaturalism 'insofar as we are dealing with etiology. . . .'[46] Foster cites as an example Latin American societies whose traditional etiologies he classifies as 'largely' naturalistic. 'In Tzintzuntzan, for example, in many hours of recording ideas about origins and cures of illness, not once has religion been mentioned – even though most villagers, if asked, would certainly agree that illness ultimately comes from God.'[47] The votive offerings of Latin Americans to Christ, the Virgin Mary, or powerful saints are not to the agents of disease but to 'merciful advocates who, if moved, can intervene to help a human sufferer'.[48]

As indicated earlier, it is impossible to discuss ethnomedicine in Lalawigan without repeated references to the supernatural. Although God and the saints are most often petitioned to cure a patient, the latter may also (though rarely) be involved in the causation of sicknesses. A primary agent of illness in the village is the spirits whose origin and powers are a blending of pagan and

Christian elements. In fact, one might blame God (at least in-directly) for disease caused by the spirits for He is responsible for their earthly presence. Even a partial sampling of cures vividly documents the melding of religious, magical, and naturalistic elements. For sicknesses such as *lanti*, elements of Catholic ritual are a prominent part of therapy. Further, although several hun-dred herbs were identified as possessing curative qualities, their preparation often requires a religious sanction, e.g. 'blessing' in church or making the medicine on Good Friday, while their effi-cacy is also partly based on imitative magic. In previous publica-tions the striking similarities between many aspects of the peasant cultures of Latin America and the Philippines, both sharing Spanish conquest and Christianization, have been documented.[49] In this regard the two culture areas are starkly contrasted.

Levels of Causality

Personalistic etiologies postulate at least two levels of causality. First, there is the *efficient* cause or agent who brings disease. Second, there is the *instrumental* (or *immediate*) cause inducing sickness.[50] For example, one efficient cause of illness in Lalawigan is the spirits, while the primary, instrumental cause of afflictions they bring is invisible foreign objects 'shot' into the victim's body. Peck suggests a third level, the *final* (or *ultimate*) cause or an attempt to answer the question: ' "Why did *this* happen to *me* at *this time* ?" '[51] According to Foster, 'Naturalistic etiologies differ significantly in that the levels of causation are much less apparent; in most cases they tend to be collapsed.'[52]

To summarize, environmental spirits, ancestral souls, and sor-cerers are the efficient causes of most serious illnesses of Lalawig-nons. The primary instrumental causes are the magic intrusion of foreign objects and the virulent 'pets' of the *barangan* and *sig-binan*. The final or ultimate cause is that the individual (or some-times a kinsman) has disturbed the invisible domain of the spirits, antagonized ancestral souls, or angered another human.[53] When they are offended or treated disrespectfully all these agents – spirits, souls, and sorcerers – retaliate with sickness (the last often at the paid request of others). Spirits and ancestral souls demand the same deference and obedience Lalawignons extend to older, wiser, richer, or more influential persons. For souls, death ends their mortal lives but not their relationships with living kinsmen.

These several distinctive levels of causality are blurred or 'collapsed' when naturalistic etiologies are examined. For example, they are obscured as explanations for sickness associated with humoral imbalances. 'Although it can be argued that a person who wilfully or through carelessness engages in activities known to upset his bodily equilibrium is the efficient cause of his illness, in practice this line of argument has little analytical value.'[54] The etiology of *lanti,* another major disease syndrome in Lalawigan, is a more complex example. Here it does not seem sensible to identify the child, who accidentally frightens himself, as the efficient cause. The agent of fright may be a parent whose experience results in the child's *lanti.* The agent's act is not purposeful as in the efficient causes for personalistic etiologies. The instrumental cause of *lanti* is fright, it is psychic and differs from the material magical missiles or 'pets' of the spirits and sorcerers. As for the ultimate cause of *lanti,* most patients are infants who would not ask this question.

As argued earlier, if one were to classify the disease etiologies of Lalawignons as either essentially personalistic or essentially naturalistic, the first system would be the obvious choice. However, some etiologies lend themselves more to arrangement on a continuum than to placement in a dichotomy. Table 2 presents disease etiologies that were chosen to illustrate their 'shading' from totally personalistic to totally naturalistic. Finally, since some diseases have multiple causes their origins must be classified as sometimes personalistic and sometimes naturalistic.

Shaman, Other Curers and Diagnosis

According to Foster personalistic etiologies 'logically require curers with supernatural and/or magical skills, for the primary concern of the patient and his family is not the immediate cause of illness, but rather "Who?" and "Why?" '[55] After his diagnosis, the curer may administer treatment or turn the patient over to another healer. In explaining his dual taxonomy for non-Western medical systems, Foster continues by stating that:

Personalistic and naturalistic etiological systems divide along

TABLE 2

Various Disease Etiologies in Barrio Lalawigan

Diseases	Causes
Epilepsy (*Buntag*)	1) Poor blood circulation; 2) inheritance; 3) environmental spirits; or 4) sorcery.
Insanity (*Mara-ot et ulo,* bad head)	1) Failure to care for oneself during menses; 2) environmental spirits; 3) St Antonio; or 4) inheritance.
Dysentery (*Disenteriya*)	1) Overeating, especially during summer when fruit is abundant (starts as diarrhoea); 2) become hot and then immediately chilled; 3) 'thorns shot' by environmental spirits into body; or 4) failure to take daily bath.
Beri-beri (*Beri-beri*)	Caused by imbalance of 'hot' and 'cold' elements in patient's body. Three varieties: 1) *beri-beri ha ginhawa* (internal, with swelling of abdomen; when it reaches the heart, death usually occurs); 2) *beri-beri ha tol-an* (bones); and 3) *beri-beri ha panit* (skin). The first variety may also cause the second and third varieties.
Tuberculosis (*Tesis*)	Typical ailment of a *tabardilio,* a person who misses meals, eats irregularly, or neglects a cold. Also through inheritance.
Asthma (*Hicab*)	May occur when phlegm in lungs of newborn child is not immediately removed; such an infant always has a cold, coughs, and eventually develops asthma. Also through inheritance.
Scabies (*Katol*)	Caused by ant bites that child infects by scratches. *Katol nga oga* (dry scabies) is caused by a tiny insect.
Malaria (*Malaria*)	1) Occurs during cold (rainy) period; and 2) some say caused by mosquito bites.
Smallpox (*Pandok*)	Once believed to be caused by environmental spirits but now believe that the cause is germs.

still another axis, the nature of the diagnosis. In personalistic systems, the shaman or witch doctor diagnoses by means of trance, or other divinatory techniques. Diagnosis – to find out who and why – is the primary skill that the patient seeks from his curer. Treatment of the instrumental cause, while important, is of secondary concern. In contrast, in naturalistic systems diagnosis is of very minor importance, as far as the curer is concerned. Diagnosis usually is made, not by the curer, but by the patient or members of his family. When the patient ceases treatment with home remedies and turns to a professional, he believes he knows what afflicts him. His primary concern is treatment to cure him.[56]

In summary, Foster believes that the 'primary role of the shaman or the witch doctor [in personalistic systems] is diagnostic, while in naturalistic systems it is *therapeutic*.'[57] With this introduction, and before an assessment is made for Lalawigan of any other aspects of the taxonomy, we examine first the various curers in the village and their basic diagnostic techniques.

The barriofolk of Lalawigan had available thirty-two folk healers practising eleven different specialities. It is these curers who diagnose and/or treat most of their major illnesses. Table 3 lists their categories, their sex, and medical specialities. Among the thirty-two healers in Lalawigan the four most common categories of curers were the *parahilot, partera, paratubod,* and *parabirik.* Healers in all but two of these four categories limited their practice primarily to diagnosing and treating *lanti.* As Table 4 indicates, one-half of all the curers in Lalawigan specialized in only one type of illness; additionally 80 per cent of the curers were female.[59]

The Shaman: Tambalan

Among the most important curers in Lalawigan are the general practitioners. These are shaman known as *tambalan* (*tambal,* to cure) or *paragbulong* (one who cures). They are noninspirational shaman whose supernatural helpers communicate with them without possession.[60] None of these shaman was an epileptic, practised self-hypnosis, or had any visible personality disorder. They were all respected members of the community. There are three ways to become a shaman: 1) selection by an ancestral soul; 2) selection by an environmental spirit; or 3) finding a magic book

TABLE 3

Curers and Their Medical Specialities in Lalawigan: 1956

Name	Sex	Primary Medical Speciality
Tambalan	Either male or female	General Practitioner
Paratubod	Female	*Lanti*
Paralo-on	Mainly female	*Lanti*
Parabirik	Female	*Lanti*
Parahaplas	Either male or female	*Barang* and *turok, to-onay,* or *hangin,* extracting foreign objects, etc. Also skin diseases caused by polluted water
Parangiho	Either male or female	Extraction of teeth
Parahilot	Mainly female	Massage, treating sprains, setting fractures, etc.
Partera	Mainly female	Pregnancy and post-natal care of mother and infant
Sunahan [58]	Either male or female	Poisonous bites
Parabadak	Either male or female	Treating *grano* boils and carbuncles
Paragabat	Either male or female	Extracting foreign objects (*hangin*)

TABLE 4

Number of Curers and Their Medical Specialities in Lalawigan: 1956

Number of Curers	Number of Medical Specialities
17	1
7	2
4	3
4	4
Totals 32	

that instructs in the art of healing. None of the four shaman (two men and two women) in Lalawigan had received their medical knowledge and skills in the third way.

The case history of one female shaman in Lalawigan is typical of shaman who receive their powers from an ancestral soul. She was twenty-eight years old when the soul of her parental great-grandfather appeared to her in a dream – 'My eyes were closed but my mind was awake.' She initially refused to accept the responsibilities of a shaman and soon after became sickly. Her parents urged her to become a shaman, otherwise she would never recover. One night she dreamed that on awakening the next morning she would find a citrus-like fruit (*tabolili*) by her sleeping mat. She was told to eat the fruit and then put the peelings on top of her head that was to be wrapped in a cloth. The next morning she found the fruit, obeyed the instructions, and was quickly cured.

In a series of subsequent dreams her great-grandfather's soul returned and instructed her on how to diagnose and cure many illnesses, describing the different herbs to use, their preparation, etc. However, she still remained both suspicious and apprehensive about accepting the call.[61] Additional dreams and the finding of unusual objects in the house occurred until she was convinced. She demanded that her great-grandfather meet her in church to seal the pact. During mass he made the sign of the cross on her right hand with a finger wet with his saliva. 'I never saw my great-grandfather again.'

The case history of one of the most active and respected male shaman in Lalawigan begins when he was ten years old. He was visited in a dream by Kagaskas who claimed to be the 'founder' of the village. Kagaskas urged him to become a shaman, promising that he would tell him how to diagnose illnesses and cure the sick. However, he was required to go to the cemetery at midnight. 'Since I was very young I did not go.' Kagaskas continued to visit the informant in his dreams over the years, leaving bottles of medicine in the house. He too finally agreed to become a shaman. In the beginning 'Kagaskas kept encouraging me for sometimes I did not cure my patients.'[62]

A third female shaman was 'visited' in her dreams by an environmental spirit who invited her to become a curer. She refused. But when her younger brother suddenly died she agreed. The spirit gave her the usual instructions for diagnosing and treating various sicknesses, assigned her a 'territory between [the towns of] San Julian and Llorente' and told her not to accept any payment except food for her services.

In the past most curers in Lalawigan were reluctant to accept payment for their medical services. 'In some instances the patient or his kinsmen demand that the curer accept a voluntary fee – usually a small sum of money, food or drink. Informants claim that the [*lanti*] rites are ineffective unless the curer is paid. However, one *lanti* curer insisted she had successfully treated many patients without being paid: "God cures without payments so why should not I?"'[63] By 1977, perhaps in response to the steady inflation of prices since 1956, most curers accepted a small money payment for their services.

Informants claim that shaman who receive their power (*gahum*) from ancestral souls practise longer than those who are assisted by the spirits. Eventually, the spirits desert their shaman. Then, since constant consultation with the spirits is required for effective diagnosis and treatment, they are forced to stop seeing patients. Moreover, the spirits may demand 'favours', not asked by the ancestral souls, that the shaman must grant. Informants told of individuals who had been offered supernatural healing powers by a spirit but who had rejected the gift. This is because the spirits always demanded a sacrifice, usually of the life of their spouse or children. In 1977 none of the shaman practising in Lalawigan claimed their powers to cure the ill were obtained from a spirit.

The third way to become a shaman is to find a magic book (*majica blanco* or white magic) that some feel was originally the property of Jesuits. The book may be found mysteriously beside one's sleeping mat on awakening, in the river or the sea, or purchased from its owner. No informants had seen such a marvellous book, but many had heard stories about them. Any shaman who depends on such a book can treat illness but not diagnose its cause. His cures are limited to remedies listed in the book once the disease's etiology is known.[64]

With the exception just noted, shaman both diagnose and treat illnesses. The most important diagnostic technique of the Lalawigan shaman is interpreting pulse beats taken at the wrist (the most important location), temples, and back of the heel. The tempo of the pulse beat tells the shaman the cause of the sicknesses, if the ailment is 'hot' or 'cold', etc. The curer also interviews the patient, enquiring about his activities in the immediate past: has he been in the forest? quarrelled with a relative or friend? had any unusual experiences, etc.? All shaman were also well-versed in the use of herbal remedies. Divination is rarely used in diagnosing illnesses, trance never.[65]

Shaman in many societies claim they are reluctant (sometimes coerced) to accept their responsibilities as curers. Filipino shaman are no exception to this general rule. For example, Lalawigan shaman must do 'penance' for their powers. Many of these behavioural and dietary restrictions occur before and during Holy Week.[66]

The Midwife: Partera

The midwife is not described in detail in this chapter for several reasons. First, the two curers most fully described in the literature for the Philippines are the shaman and midwife.[67] Second, an extensive account of the midwife in a Cebuan Bisayan village (Caticugan) in Negros Islands has been published.[68] The *partera* in Lalawigan shares many beliefs and practices reported for the midwife in Caticugan, with one drastic exception. The midwives in Lalawigan do not claim their knowledge and skills are of supernatural origin. They were taught when young by other *parteras*, usually a parent or another older relative. The midwife begins her care of a pregnant woman several months after conception, continues it through pregnancy, delivery, and into the post-delivery period. The *partera* is both the village obstetrician and pediatrician.

Most informants claimed that in the past nearly all midwives were men. They were sought because of their greater strength, especially for difficult deliveries. During residence in the village in 1956 some *parteras* were male. In 1977 one of these male midwives was still living but no longer delivered. At present all practising midwives in Lalawigan are females.

Sunahan

Sunahan specialize in diagnosing and treating poisonous bites (*sunugod*) of insects (spiders, centipedes, etc.), snakes, and punctures (*nahitunok*) by fish with venomous fins. They also treat *sigbin* bites (*tenucob hin sigbin*). The treatment is called *suna*. The only *sunahan* practising in Lalawigan during residence was also a *tambalan*. In 1977 only one *sunahan* lived in Lalawigan, and he was not a *tambalan*. Informants, and the *sunahan*, claimed there were three types of this variety of healer: those (1) whose knowledge and remedies came originally from a twin who was a snake; (2) who treated bites only with saliva, unaccompanied by prayers; and (3) who used various herbal remedies and prayers. In 1977 both of the two *sunahan* practising in the locality (one each in Lalawigan and Borongan) had an ancestor who had a twin snake. This power was transmitted to direct descendants to the seventh generation. By sucking the wound one Lalawigan *sunahan* (1956), who used herbs and prayers, could identify the poisonous snake that had bitten a patient. 'Some snake bites are sour while others are bitter or sweet.' He said that when a person is bitten by a poisonous snake, the *sunahan's* mouth immediately becomes unusually dry. Sometimes the snake bite is lanced before herbs are applied: 'When I do this the bite may "smoke" because of the poison.' [69]

Parangiho

The *parangiho* (*ngiho*, to pull or to extract) extracts decayed teeth by slowly rocking the tooth with his fingers while reciting a secret prayer. No one hears the prayer because the '*parangiho* recites it so softly one cannot understand it.' If the patient is frightened, the extraction is stopped for the 'person will become ill.' After an extraction, the patient gargles with 'blessed' vinegar. Some informants believe it is unwise to have teeth extracted in this manner since the other teeth will loosen and soon require removal too. This specialist learns how to extract teeth from another *parangiho*.

Parahilot

It is not surprising to find that the *parahilot*, whose primary skill is massage, is the most numerous of all curers in Lalawigan. The

moist, damp climate and the types of clothing and residences con-
spire to make aches and pains in the joints and muscles common,
especially among older people. *Parahilot* skills as curers are taught
to their children or other young kinsmen. For example, one *parahilot* said his father taught him how to massage: 'We were always
together, I even slept with him.' This curer also uses various herbal
remedies.

Parahilot who were breech births (*sohi*) have the inborn ability
to remove obstructions (*bukog*, especially fish bones) lodged in the
throat. Several but not all of these curers in Lalawigan were breech
births. One *sohi parahilot* remembered that 'When I was small I
was dragged to help a person with a fish bone stuck in his throat. I
rubbed my hand across his throat. There must be some power in
my hand because I was successful even though I was small and did
it against my will.' The folk logic is that individuals who were
abnormally located within their mother's womb yet were born
alive can extract objects lodged abnormally in the throat. *Sohi
parahilot* are considered the best of all *parahilot*.

Parahaplas

There were only two *parahaplas* (brother and sister) in Lalawigan.
They had learned their skills from kinsmen when young. Neither
of them limited their practice to *haplas*. Their treatment, as described earlier, was not restricted to anointing as done by their
counterparts in Guinhangdan.

In summary, most patients seek healers in Lalawigan either for
diagnosis and treatment of serious ailments or solely for treatment
(if the etiology has been determined earlier). Rarely does a seriously ill patient go to a curer solely for diagnosis. As the preceding
section on curers indicates, many are specialists whose diagnostic
skills are innate (e.g. *sohi parahilot*) or esoteric (e.g. *tambalan*).
Finally the use of trance or divination in diagnosis is rare in this
community. An incomplete survey of the literature on the Christian Filipino suggests, however, that divination as a means of
diagnosis may be more common in the Philippines than indicated
by its rarity in Lalawigan.[70] In conclusion, Foster's taxonomy for

personalistic-naturalistic systems of etiologies does not fully apply to the curers of Lalawigan whose treatment of the instrumental cause of illness is as important as their identification of its efficient cause. The major role of the shaman and most other curers, for the predominantly personalistic etiological system of Lalawigan, is to act both as a diagnostician and therapeutician.

Preventive Medicine

Foster's 'highly impressionistic' opinion is that preventive medicine in naturalistic etiologies correlates predominantly with 'don'ts', while 'do's' are emphasized in personalistic etiologies.[71] In naturalistic systems the individual, to maintain his health, avoids situations or behaviour that result in illness. Personalistic systems stress that good health is the result of successfully reaching out for harmonious relationships with supernaturals, kinsmen, and neighbours.

> Although this means avoiding those acts known to arouse resentment–'don'ts'–it particularly means careful attention being paid to the propitiatory rituals that are a god's due, to positive demonstrations to ancestors that they have not been forgotten, and to friendly acts to neighbors and fellow villagers that remind them that their good will is valued.[72]

The 'do's' appear to predominate personal health strategies of Lalawignons, although there are also the 'don'ts'. Numerous illnesses are interpreted as the result of antagonizing the environmental spirits, ancestral souls, or sorcerers. As in Latin America, many major sicknesses that afflict Lalawignons can be avoided if 'one's social networks, with fellow human beings, with ancestors, and with deities, are maintained in good working order'.[73]

Another factor in preventive medicine, not mentioned by Foster, is charms, since reliance on them may be 'physically hygienic'.[74] They can be regarded as 'do's'. (Charms were not a major research topic in Lalawigan, but scattered information was gathered). Arens studied charms in some detail, with most of his informants coming from the Samaran cultural-linguistic area. He proposed that charms be divided into two categories, amulets and talismans.

The reason for the distinction between amulet and talisman lies in the folk belief that amulets have preventive force against witchcraft, sickness, accidents, and the like, whereas talismans bring good luck or transmit new qualities.[75]

This general distinction between amulets and talismans was found valid by Scheans and Hutterer in their investigation of tattooed charms in Samar. Arens cautions, however, that this distinction cannot be maintained in all instances, e.g. some amulets also are said to bring the wearer good luck.

The common name for amulet, in Lalawigan and other Samaran localities, is *sumpa,* meaning to protect oneself from being 'overpowered' by supernatural entities and sorcerers. A popular name for talisman is *sangod,* best translated as a good-luck charm.[76] Some specific powers of the various amulets are to heal wounds, protect the wearer against poisoning, ensure a normal delivery, guard a child against *lanti,* ward off sicknesses caused by the spirits and sorcerers, etc. Amulets are usually worn only by children in Lalawigan since their health is more difficult to maintain than that of adults and they are most frequently the victims of the spirits. These amulets were often a small red cloth packet or empty bullet case, filled with magical items, and hung around the neck or pinned to the clothing. Inside the charm may be put a herb recommended by the shaman, an *oracion,* small crucifix, etc. Some contained a scrap of paper on which Latin words were written.[77] Amulets and talismans are purchased in the Borongan marketplace, supplied by the *tambalan,* or are bought from itinerant peddlers who pass through the barrio, e.g. a crocodile's tooth. Catholic medallions are also worn. A gold or diamond ring is also believed to be an effective amulet.[78] These charms are usually inexpensive, although one family reputedly paid fifty pesos (in 1956 about $25 US) for an anti-*barang* amulet.

Not only the individual but his residence may be protected by amulets. The most common household *sumpa* in Lalawigan is the *asugi (asugui).* About one-half of the residences in Lalawigan had an *asugi,* often hung near the door or a window. The *asugi* was believed especially effective in guarding the occupants of the house from *sigbin* bites. Arens' informants also named the *asugi* as an excellent protection from the spirits. *Asugi* are small glass bottles filled with mercury, moss and pebbles, the latter often being silver or gold in colour. The mercury in the bottle contains small oily bubbles called *asugi*. These bubbles are alive; they multiply constantly if most of the liquid is drained each Friday or on sorrowful days of the Catholic religious calendar.[79] Finally, crossing oneself is a common practice when leaving the dwelling. It is regarded as a preventative charm against a supernatural attack that might otherwise result in sickness and injury.

There are also 'do's' for maintaining good health such as taking a daily bath, maintaining the 'hot' and 'cold' equilibrium of the body, not bathing immediately if one has been working under a hot sun, not eating fruits or sweets before breakfast, not bathing while menstruating, etc.

There are numerous tabus (*maglihi* or *lihi*) whose violation is said to result in illness, abnormal mental behaviour, or to affect an unborn child. Tabus often are associated with pregnancy or prenatal influences. Not all Lalawignons believe in every tabu; indeed some tabus appear to be known to only a few people. Yet most of the barriofolk believe it is unwise to violate many tabus – 'It does not cost anything to be careful.'

An analysis of the tabus associated with pregnancy in the Philippines has been published elsewhere.[80] The four emphases of tabus that this analysis identifies also occur in Lalawigan. First, there are dietary prohibitions. These tabus are fewer in number than are behavioural restrictions and are not predominantly hygienic. Second, some restrictions are genuinely prophylactic, e.g. limiting excessive carbohydrate and salt intake during pregnancy. Third, the tabus reflect two basic concerns of a pregnant Filipina: the act of delivery and the physical condition of the infant. Fourth, they refute the popular belief in most societies that pregnancy and childbirth are casual and non-threatening events resulting in only a slight disruption of the mother's usual duties.

The Locus of Responsibility

Foster asserts that two etiological systems (personalistic and naturalistic) also differ in regard to an individual's responsibility for his sickness. For naturalistic etiologies 'the exercise of absolute care in avoiding disease-producing situations should, in theory, keep one healthy. Hence, illness is *prima facie* evidence that the patient has been guilty of lack of care.'[81] For the other system Foster notes:

> But personalistic causality is far more complex than naturalistic causality, since there are no absolute rules to avoid arousing the envy of others, for doing just the right amount of ritual to satisfy an ancestor, for knowing how far one can shade a taboo without actually breaching it. Consequently, in such systems one has less control over the conditions that lead to illness than in the other [naturalistic], where the rules are clearly stated.[82]

The preceding data for Lalawigan illustrate how relatively limited is the control the individual exerts over many causes of sickness. To exist one must fish, farm, cut trees in the forest, graze animals, and interact with kinsmen, friends, and strangers. All these activities may, often unknowingly and unintentionally, antagonize the environmental spirits or offend a sorcerer (or someone who hires him). It is equally impossible to ensure that one's every act is agreeable to the ancestral souls whose core of values is unchanging and conservative.[83] This is not to imply, as this chapter documents, that Lalawignons lack all control over situations causing sickness. Yet careful observance of 'naturalistic' rules for good health is not enough to protect one from illness.

Conclusion

The application of Foster's taxonomy to the disease etiologies of Lalawignons indicates that they fall primarily into the personalistic category. It is hypothesized that the personalistic model is typical of the disease etiologies of other Christian Filipino cultural-linguistic groups. For example, the Nydeggers report that 'By far the greatest number of illnesses, accidents, and deaths are attributed to the *not-humans* [environmental spirits].'[84] One major difference is that the Lalawigan shaman (and probably typical for Filipino shaman in general) has broader medical functions than those Foster assigns this curer for personalistic systems in general.

Perhaps the most important reason most curers in Lalawigan both diagnose and treat illness is that their procedures usually require specialized knowledge and skills, some 'inherited' or innate. Since illness is frequently interpreted as of supernatural origin, specialists are required to determine the exact preternatural agent, e.g. whether the spirits, ancestral souls, etc. Once the etiology is known, treatment is often complicated for it may demand extensive knowledge of herbal remedies, exoteric rituals, etc. The average Lalawignon, lacking this specialized knowledge, would probably be apprehensive, for example, that a ritual improperly done might worsen not cure the sickness. Another reason, possibly more important in the past than today, is that the fee for consulting a traditional curer, when paid, was small (usually a token gift of food or drink) and covered both diagnosis and cure.

Some refinement of Foster's personalistic-naturalistic taxonomy is desirable. First, amulets and talismans should be added to the preventive medicines as a diagnostic characteristic. Second, in numerous societies it is impossible to put some diseases into a single category. Others have written that a disease may be assigned different etiologies by various individuals in the same community.[85] The traditional categories of supernaturally and naturally caused diseases have recognized limitations. Ackerknecht has argued that some medical beliefs and practices are neither supernatural nor natural in origin, but *habitual.* 'Tradition determines certain almost automatic acts in certain situations. . . . To call such attitudes "naturalistic" or "rational" seems to inject into the data contents they actually do not have. People in this case operate below the threshold of full consciousness.'[86] However, his habitual category has not been widely adopted by medical anthropologists.

For the Philippines Lieban divides etiologies into natural and supernatural.[87] Jocano separates disease etiologies for his Tagalog area into three classes: supernatural, natural, and innate. Innate disorders are those illnesses traced to heredity, psychic experiences (auditory, visual, haptic, and mephitic phenomena), blood composition, etc. However, his own detailed and excellent account of folk medicine indicates this scheme is not entirely satisfactory. Finally, the same affliction may be blamed on different causes among Filipino groups. Mental disorders that Jocano classifies as of innate origin for Tagalogs are blamed on both natural and supernatural etiologies among Cebuan Filipinos, e.g. heredity, spirits, sorcery, etc.[88]

Third, the etiology of a disease may be assigned an efficient cause that is supernatural, while the instrumental cause is believed natural. For example, among some Mexican-Americans witchcraft may be considered the source of sickness but germs are the instrumental cause,[89] and among the Azande, where a burn is believed to be caused by scalding water, the accident is also seen as the result of witchcraft.[90] For one Tagalog community a naturally caused disease may later be categorized as of supernatural origin if the patient does not respond to treatment.[91] Gould found in India that various informants gave different etiologies to the same disease. Since the symptoms of a disease varied, it was impossible to assign it a single slot in the precise classification scheme he proposed in an earlier publication.[92] This same theme is discussed by Bidney as the principle of multiple etiology that denies there is a final efficient cause for any single illness.[93]

Future researchers should heed Fabrega's recommendation that attention be given to the 'Presumed sources of types of ultimate causes that are attributed to the illness in its *various stages* [emphasis added].'[94] It would be wise to get various informants to discuss each case for they may offer different interpretations of its causes.[95] These varying factors could, in some societies, significantly influence the classification of an etiological system as either personalistic or naturalistic, depending on the selection of one of several etiologies assigned to various diseases.

NOTES AND REFERENCES

1   This research was done when the author had a Fulbright Research Fellowship to the Philippines. He acknowledges the superb co-operation of the Philippine-American Educational Foundation (Fulbright) in Manila and the skilled ongoing assistance received from his research associate in eastern Samar, Mr Felipe Dala. Information in this chapter for 1977 was obtained by Mr Dala at the author's request. Drafts of this manuscript have profited from the criticisms of Fred Eggan, George Foster, Morton Netzorg, and Ronald Provencher. The language of Filipinos living in eastern Leyte and Samar has also been called *Waray-waray* ('Nothing-nothing') or Lineyte-Samarnon.

2   Although considerable ethnographical detail (and variations) has been omitted from this account, some illustrative examples are given in the footnotes. Most references (often without giving any comparative content) are limited to the literature on ethnomedicine among Samaran Filipinos. How-

ever, for comparative purposes, references are made to the numerous and perceptive publications on traditional medicine by Richard Lieban, although his research pertains to Cebuan Filipinos in Negros Oriental Province and Cebu City, Cebu.

3　Donn V. Hart, 'Christian Filipinos', in Frank M. LeBar (ed.), *Ethnic Groups of Insular Southeast Asia,* New Haven, Conn., HRAF Press, Vol. 2, 1975, pp. 16-22.

4　George M. Foster, 'Disease etiologies in non-Western medical systems', *American Anthropologist,* Vol. 78, 1976, p. 775.

5　The *maglimbunganon* greeted the first Spaniards to set foot on the Philippines in the sixteenth century. These spirits are now regarded as humans ousted from heaven because they refused baptism. One popular and widespread explanation of their origin is that one day when God (or St Peter) was absent from heaven, Rosbel (the brother of St Michael) or Lucifer sprinkled holy water on the ground. Each drop miraculously became a human with supernatural powers. When God returned to heaven He insisted that these newly-created people be baptized to remain in heaven. The priest in the Philippines, during a christening, puts a pinch of salt on the child's tongue as a symbol of the preservation of the faith. This action or principle of imitative magic was interpreted differently by the unbaptized persons in heaven. They reasoned that as salt vanishes in water, baptism would result in the immediate loss of their supernatural powers. They refused baptism. In retaliation God spent forty days and nights sweeping heaven of these ingrates who 'fell to the earth like rain', dropping upon the ocean, land, forest, rivers, springs, etc. Sometimes the environmental spirits are also referred to as *panolay,* demons who have horns and tails, live in hell and are under the authority of *Yawa* (a contraction of Yaweh) or Lucifer. The *panolay* fell from heaven directly into hell, while the environment spirits landed on the earth and sea. Since they may roam the earth, deceiving people, the *panolay* are also *maglimbunganon.* For a similar version for Samarans see Villegas, note 14. These spirits are known elsewhere in the Philippines as *anitos, ingkantos* (*encantos,* from the Spanish *encantar,* to enchant).

6　For an extensive account of the rituals associated with the *dagatnon* and *lawodnon,* see Richard Arens, SVD, 'Animistic fishing rituals in Leyte and Samar', *Leyte-Samar Studies,* Vol. 4, 1971, pp. 42-7. Originally published in *The Philippine Sociological Review,* Vol. 4, 1956, pp. 24-8.

7　The most powerful *dalakitnon* live in the balete tree known as *kalumpang,* next in power are those residing in the *tabas* balete. The *dalakitnon* living in the *momhanay* balete are relatively harmless and may assist humans if treated respectfully.

8　The male *agta* has a fin down his spine. When he moves rapidly he makes a slapping noise caused by his large testes hitting his inner thighs. *Agta* are fond of stealing chickens (only to eat their eyes) but can be scared away by the beam of a flashlight. Arens, op. cit., p. 25, reports that the *agta* in Leyte (Cebuan-speaking regions?) are believed to be small people, while in Samar they are 'big, tall, and black' (1971a:20,25).

9   Donn V. Hart, 'The Filipino villager and his spirits', *Solidarity,* Vol. 1, 1966, p. 68.

10   Numerous signs identify where some spirits live. For example, the *pokdao* is a tree or rock formation (on land or sea) that 'looks like a human'. The formation is regarded as a sign that the 'spot is enchanted'. Although they grow in size they never move. They are considered 'alive' for a *pokdao* tree bleeds when cut. One woodcutter died ('His body looked like it was burned') when he tried to cut such a tree. In fact, it is said to be impossible to fell a *pokdao* tree for 'it does not fall to the ground when cut but merely spins.'

11   Lieban makes the identical statement about the spirits (*ingkanto*) for the Cebuans of eastern Negros Island. Richard Lieban, 'The dangerous Ingkantos: illness and social control', *American Anthropologist,* Vol. 64, 1962, p. 309.

12   Usually the *katig-uban* is directed by a female who specializes in Catholic folk ritual, e.g. *parapamatbat* (*pamatbat,* to lead a prayer) or a *padi-padi* (priest-priest, i.e., not a real priest). When a food offering is made it includes all common items in the diet. Cooked food is not seasoned with salt, for salted dishes are anathema to both the spirits and souls. Some families hold their annual ritual after the harvest (when food is plentiful) or co-ordinate it with the annual fiesta when food preparations are elaborate and most families entertain visiting kinsmen and friends. The offering in the past sometimes included a roast pig, minus its head and legs, covered with its own fat. On the pig's back is traced an outline of the *halo* lizard. Sometimes the pig's head is placed on a rice winnowing basket, surrounded by rice cakes. The participants consider the food as 'eaten' by the souls when the *halo* lizard makes its customary sound.

13   Another involvement of the souls in curing is that on occasions food is placed on the residential altar as an offering to one's deceased ancestors. Later this 'blessed' food (the offering is accompanied by prayers) is fed to a patient for its curative qualities.

14   The *barangan,* whose powers and activities vary, is discussed in other sources for Leyte and Samar. See Ethel Nurge, 'Etiology of illness in Guin-hangdan', *American Anthropologist,* Vol. 60, 1958, pp. 1158-72; and Sister Maria G. Villegas, R.S.M., 'Superstitious beliefs and practices in the coastal towns of eastern Leyte', *Leyte-Samar Studies,* Vol. 2, 1968, pp. 221-32.

15   For a more detailed description of the *barangan,* including data from eastern Samar, see Richard Arens, SVD, 'The *Tambalan* and his medical practices in Leyte and Samar Islands', *Leyte-Samar Studies,* Vol. 4, 1971, pp. 107-21. Originally published in *The Philippine Journal of Science,* Vol. 85, 1957, pp. 121-30.

16   The only effective sources of medicinal coconut oil are the first reddish-brown coconuts borne by a young tree or the only nut facing east on the tree. The oil (which can be extracted from the meat only on Good Friday) is poured into a bottle containing various herbs and a piece of coral. Some

herbs used are *puti* (the roots of a tall grass whose name also means white), *manawog* (a black sea plant), seeds of the *tangantangan* tree, and coral called *dalakit ha lawod* (balete of the sea). Herbal materials for curative purposes often are secured from the eastern side of a plant or tree, the direction the sun rises, hence 'rising' or improving the patient's condition. Items are also gathered from the western side of a plant, the direction the sun sets, when they are used to 'sink' or induce illness.

17   One shaman used a medicinal water in which the following herbs were soaked: *balodawi* (a vine similar to rattan), *tagum* (a shrub with long pointed green fruit), cogon grass roots, *bagakay* (a small thornless bamboo), and *papawran* (a tall sugar-cane-like grass similar to *talahib*). Most of the herbs grow wild, although several Lalawigan families cultivated a few popular herbs, e.g. *ganda, kusol, panigbin,* etc.

18   *Dalungdongan* also refers to the *barangan, sigbinan,* or *asuwang*. The *asuwang* is a human with preternatural powers who is particularly fond of preying on pregnant women or newly-delivered mothers.

19   Although effort was made to determine the cause of deaths supposedly due to *sigbin* bites, their actual etiology remains unknown. Another source states that *sigbins* 'are goat-like animals with big, wide and prominent ears but no horns', Richard Arens, SVD, 'Witches and witchcraft in Leyte and Samar', *Leyte-Samar Studies*, Vol. 5, 1971, p. 92. Originally published in *The Philippine Journal of Science,* Vol. 85, 1956, pp. 451-65.

20   The curer smuggles vinegar (*suka nga inorasion*) and medicinal coconut oil into church in a small bottle under his clothing. During mass he tries to stand close to the priest so the fluid is 'blessed'.

21   Space prohibits listing the herbal remedies, but some common herbs used to treat a *sigbin* bite are: *panigbin, ganda, tol-anmanok* (also meaning chicken bone), *amor seco, amomonti, puti papawran,* and *makaranas.* The last two herbs are grasses. Leaves from the *manban* bush, new abaca suckers, leaves of the *tabolilid* and *kalamansi* trees, and *tisa* are also utilized.

22   See also Nurge, op. cit., p. 1166.

23   F. Landa Jocano, *Folk Medicine in a Philippine Municipality: An Analysis of the System of Folk Healing in Bay, Laguna, and Its Implications for the Introduction of Modern Medicine,* Manila, The National Museum, 1973, p. 32.

24   One story in a supplementary reader, approved for use in the public elementary schools, is about birds attending a class where the teacher is a parrot. One pupil, the hawk, claims she does not believe in God. Later the hawk returns to school, lamenting that all her children are sick. She has consulted many physicians without success. The parrot tells her pupils to pray to God for the recovery of the hawk's babies. Since the sick children are cured, the hawk is convinced that God exists. Trinidad Sion, *The Little Chicks and Other Stories,* Manila, 1949.

25   Richard Lieban, 'Fatalism and medicine in Cebuano areas of the Philippines', *Anthropological Quarterly,* Vol. 39, 1966, p. 174.

26 Lee Sechrest, 'Conceptions and management of mental disorder in some Negros oriental barrios', *Philippine Sociological Review*, Vol. 18, 1970, p. 8.

27 Nurge, op. cit., p. 1165.

28 Richard Lieban, *Cebuano Sorcery: Malign Magic in the Philippines*, Berkeley, University of California Press, 1967, p. 33.

29 Younger people can (extremely rarely) cause *gaba* to older people. When this occurs the curse is more dangerous for 'what older person can kneel to a younger person, requesting his forgiveness?'

30 Foster, op. cit., p. 776.

31 The *katao* is a 'merperson' (half-human and half-fish) who lives in the sea. One fisherman in another village was believed to have been befriended by a *katao*: 'He became rich.' However, when his house burned to the ground, the people believed the *katao* had deserted him. Lalawigan fishermen report hearing the sounds of animals (cows, chickens, quail, etc.) that belong to the *katao* coming from under the sea. A strand of *katao* beard is a good-luck fishing charm (*sangod*). Drowned fishermen whose bodies are not recovered are believed to become slaves of the *katao*.

32 Erwin H. Ackerknecht, 'Primitive medicine', *Transactions, N.Y. Academy of Sciences* (Series II), Vol. 8, 1945, pp. 27-8; and A. Irving Hallowell, 'The social function of anxiety in a primitive society', *American Sociological Review*, Vol. 6, 1941, pp. 264-5.

33 Richard Lieban, 'Medical Anthropology', in John J. Honigmann (ed.), *Handbook of Social and Cultural Anthropology*, Chicago, Rand McNally College Publishing Company, 1973, p. 1049.

34 Foster, op. cit., p. 774.

35 Ibid., p. 775.

36 Ibid.

37 Donn V. Hart, *Bisayan Filipino and Malayan Humoral Pathologies: Folk Medicine and Ethno-history in Southeast Asia*, Southeast Asian Program, Data Paper No. 76, Ithaca, New York, Cornell University, 1969.

38 Ibid., p. 71.

39 Ibid., p. 80.

40 It might be noted that the 'hot-cold' syndrome in Latin America has been extended to a world view (see W. Madsen, 'Hot and cold in the universe of San Francisco Tecospa, Valley of Mexico', *Journal of American Folklore*, Vol. 68, 1955, pp. 123-39) and a model of social relations (see R. L. Currier, 'The hot-cold syndrome and symbolic balance in Mexican and Spanish-American folk medicine', *Ethnology*, Vol. 5, 1966, pp. 251-63). Moreover, in some societies an imbalance of 'hot' and 'cold' elements can produce natural disasters, e.g. drought, Hart, op. cit. (1969).

41 Foster, op. cit., p. 776.

42 Since this syndrome has been discussed in another publication only a summary of *lanti* is presented. See Donn V. Hart, 'Lanti: sickness by fright:

a Bisayan Filipino peasant syndrome', *Philippine Quarterly of Culture and Society,* Vol. 3, 1975, pp. 1-19.

43 Edward Norbeck, *Religion in Primitive Society,* New York, Harper and Row, 1961, p. 56.

44 The specialists in *lanti* are known after the names of its three different treatments: *paratubod, paralo-on,* and *parabirik.* Some parents resist initiation of any *lanti* curing rite since 'It becomes a habit.' For example, one grandmother scolded her daughter for having the first *lanti* curing rite for her grandson: 'Now this treatment will be necessary in the future for his children and their descendants.'

45 Foster, op. cit., p. 777.

46 Ibid.

47 Ibid., p. 773.

48 Ibid., p. 777.

49 Donn V. Hart, *The Philippine Plaza Complex: A Focal Point in Culture Change,* New Haven, Conn., Yale University, Southeast Asia Studies, Cultural Report Series No. 3, 1955; Donn V. Hart, op. cit., (1969); Donn V. Hart, *Compadrinazgo: Ritual Kinship in the Philippines,* DeKalb, Illinois, Northern Illinois University Press, 1977.

50 Foster, op. cit., p. 778.

51 John C. Peck, 'Doctor medicine and bush medicine in Kaukira, Honduras', in Thomas Weaver (ed.), *Essays on Medical Anthropology,* Athens, Georgia, University of Georgia Press, Southern Anthropological Society Proceedings, Vol. 1, 1968, p. 78.

52 Foster, op. cit., p. 778.

53 The final cause of a *sigbin* attack is less apparent, but it seems to be that the *sigbinan's* 'pets' are hungry because their owner is a poor, lazy cannibal.

54 Foster, op. cit., p. 778.

55 Ibid.

56 Ibid., p. 779.

57 Ibid.

58 One popular *sunahan* in Lalawigan in 1977 treated *sigbin* bites with herbs and saliva, applied to the bitten part of the body. For snake or insect bites, only saliva was used. His mother, he claimed, had a snake as a twin.

59 Various factors explain this division of labour by sex among curers in Lalawigan. First, many curing procedures require extensive knowledge of formal and folk Catholicism (e.g. prayers, including novenas). This knowledge is primarily the possession of women. Women are far more active than most men in church affairs in Lalawigan. They decorate the chapel for religious events, attend mass more regularly, compose most of the members of sodalities, and organize and lead the various Catholic rituals performed before the family altar. Second, all but one of the specialists in *lanti* are females. This predominance probably reflects the fact that *lanti* is

associated almost entirely with infants and small children – who are the domestic domain of the mother. A third factor that partly explains the many female curers in Lalawigan is that these skills are usually transmitted from female to female or male to male. Finally, only a few families supplied most of the curers. Six families accounted for 19 of the 32 curers in the barrio. In one family five siblings (including one brother) were curers, while in another family six sisters represented every speciality in Lalawigan except the treatment of *grano* lesions.

Although there were two male midwives in Lalawigan, one was consulted only for difficult deliveries. Since rituals and medical skills (including use of herbs) for many illnesses are transmitted to kinsmen (parents to children, grandparents to grandchildren, etc.), one can expect most future curers in Lalawigan to be female members of a few barrio families. Lieban found that males predominated among folk curers in Cebu City (1967). All of the three midwives in Tarong were men. William F. Nydegger and Corinne Nydegger, *Tarong: An Ilocos Barrio in the Philippines,* New York, John Wiley and Sons, Inc., Six Cultures Series, Vol. 6, 1966, p. 85. They added that male midwives were not uncommon in the Ilokan region. There may be special or regional factors related to the sexual selection of curers.

60   Some might not classify these *tambalan* as shaman. See David Landy (ed.), *Culture, Disease and Healing: Studies in Medical Anthropology,* New York, Macmillan, 1977, p. 17.

61   She was unwilling, for example, to go as instructed to the cemetery to pray at midnight for nine consecutive Fridays. Finally, her great-grand-father urged her 'to try to cure my cousin' who had been bitten by a *sigbin*. 'If you fail,' he bargained, 'you do not have to be a shaman.' However, her treatment cured her cousin.

62   In another dream the informant was visited by a woman ('She was a pure Filipina') who told him to wrap his hand in a white handkerchief. When the handkerchief was removed, his hand had the 'power to cure any disease'. This woman (not an ancestor) also instructed him in how to pre-pare various herbs for treating his patients. Finally, he discovered that God (in a later interview he said it might have been his maternal grandmother who had been a shaman) had given him the gift of diagnosing illnesses by feeling a patient's pulse.

63   Hart, op. cit (1975), p. 6. See also Villegas, op. cit., p. 224.

64   One incident is reported of a man finding a similar book (of *oraciones*) while ploughing his field. The finder interpreted this discovery as a sign (later confirmed in dreams) that he was selected to become a *tambalan*. However, he also received training in healing from his paternal grandfather. Both his grandfather and father were *tambalan*. See Daniel J. Scheans and Karl Hutterer, 'Some Oracion tattoos from Samar', *Leyte-Samar Studies,* Vol. 4, 1970, pp. 30-31.

65   Some *tambalan* in this region do use divination for diagnosis and treatment of illnesses. Richard Arens, SVD, 'The use of amulets and talis-mans in Leyte and Samar', *Leyte-Samar Studies,* Vol. 5, 1971, pp. 122-3.

Originally published in *The Journal of East Asiatic Studies,* Vol. 6, 1957, pp. 115-27. (The original article includes photographs of amulets and talismans omitted in reprinting.) In this article Arens describes how one shaman tried to stand an egg on end on a bottle lying horizontally on the table. If the egg stood 'the sickness is due to some spirits of their dead ancestors who are angry because the family members have forgotten to pray for them' [Arens, op. cit. (1971), p. 109]. Arens adds that shaman in Bohol Island are reported to use a magical stone (*mutya*) to divine the cause of illness. Lieban briefly describes the use of divination by Cebuan shaman in diagnosing disease, op. cit. (1967), p. 82, and in his 'Symbols, signs, and success: healers and power in a Philippine City', in R. D. Fogelson and R. Adams (eds.), *The Anthropology of Power: Ethnographic Studies from Asia, Oceania, and the New World,* New York, Academic Press, 1977, p. 59. Divination observed in Lalawigan was limited to *lanti.* A resinous substance put in the fire slowly took the shape of the agent causing the child's fright. No healers were seen going into trance during a curing session and all interviewed denied the use of this technique. Shakman reports that five of twenty-two traditional healers interviewed by him entered a state of trance as part of the treatment process, Robert Shakman, 'Indigenous healing of mental illness in the Philippines', *The International Journal of Social Psychiatry,* Vol. 15, 1969, p. 281.

66   Some said the shaman must not speak during Holy Week. One shaman fasted on Tuesdays and Fridays six weeks before and during Holy Week. He ate meat or fish only on Sunday; the rest of the week his only food was rice and salt. However, his friends advised him not to fast so intensively since he had to work hard to support his large family. Now he fasts by skipping breakfasts on Tuesdays and Fridays during the seven-week period.

67   Nurge, op. cit.; Jocano, op. cit. (1973); and Nydegger and Nydegger, op. cit.

68   Donn V. Hart, 'From pregnancy through birth in a Filipino Bisayan village', in Donn V. Hart, Phya Anuman Rajadhon and Richard J. Coughlin, *Southeast Asian Birth Customs: Three Studies in Human Reproduction,* New Haven, Conn., Human Relations Area Files Press, 1965, pp. 1-113.

69   One of numerous herbal remedies the Lalawigan *sunahan* used for poisonous spider bites was shredded bark of the *laglag* (*paglaglag,* to kill) tree or the young fronds of the *morokporok* fern or stems of the *badyang* mixed with 'blessed' vinegar and applied as a poultice (*hapas*). All bites must be first washed with kerosene. For centipede bites he used a poultice of *laglag* roots, chewed into a spongy mass while saying a secret prayer. For snake bites he heated a deer's horn, 'as hot as the patient can stand' and applied it to the bite region. If the horn stuck, the person would recover.

70   A medical doctor who practised in rural Luzon describes eight different ways one folk curer divined the cause of illness, Juan M. Flavier, *My Friends in the Barrio,* Quezon City, New Day Publishers, 1974, pp. 88-109.

71   Foster, op. cit., p. 780.

72   Ibid.

73   Ibid.

74   Lieban, op. cit. (1973), p. 1046.

75   Arens, op. cit. (1971), pp. 122-3.

76   Other terms for amulets are *biyao, pankontra, hapin ha lawas* (covering for the body), *sob-ong, pingkit* (to pin), and *quenta* (necklace). Another name for talisman is *saot*. See also Arens, op. cit. (1971), p. 123. There are talismans for good luck in gambling, love-making, to achieve invulnerability and invisibility, etc. (Also see Villegas, op. cit., p. 224). For a discussion of charms in the Ilokan region, see Nydegger and Nydegger, op. cit., p. 76. Charms have an important role in folk medical practices in this Ilokan village.

77   Would-be Latin is used in charms and also in curing rituals. Few if any of the barriofolk know the meaning of the Latin words and phrases that are usually confused, garbled and misspelled in the process of oral transmission. It is believed, however, that God used Latin when He evicted the ancestors of the environmenal spirits from heaven. 'The spirits still hate these words because they are non-Christians.' Sometimes Latin words are written on paper that is soaked in water that the patient drinks as a medicine.

78   Villegas, op. cit., p. 231.

79   One obtains an *asugi* by getting a 'start' from a friend. Some moss is secured and put in a bottle with water. The moss supposedly generates the *asugi*. Some informants claimed the moss is the 'feces of the asugi'. Fluid from the *asugi* also has various medicinal qualities not described here.

80   Hart, op. cit. (1965).

81   Foster, op. cit., p. 780.

82   Ibid.

83   Lieban, op. cit. (1973), p. 1050.

84   Nydegger and Nydegger, op. cit., p. 73.

85   E. E. Evans-Pritchard, *Witchcraft, Oracles and Magic Among the Azande,* London, Oxford University Press, 1937, p. 129.

86   Erwin H. Ackerknecht, *Medicine and Ethnology: Selected Essays,* Baltimore, Maryland, The Johns Hopkins University Press, 1971, p. 146.

87   Lieban, op. cit. (1967), pp. 81-2.

88   Sechrest, op. cit., p. 6.

89   Margaret Clark, *Health in the Mexican-American Culture: A Community Study,* Berkeley, California, University of California Press, 1970, p. 164.

90   Evans-Pritchard, op. cit., pp. 507-8.

91   F. Landa Jocano, *The Traditional World of Malitbog,* Quezon City, University of the Philippines Press, 1969, p. 299.

92   Harold A. Gould, 'Modern medicine and folk cognition in rural india', *Human Organization,* Vol. 24, 1965, pp. 201-8.

93   David Bidney, 'So-called primitive medicine and religion', in Iago

Galdston (ed.), *Medicine and Anthropology,* New York, International Universities Press, 1963, pp. 141-56.

94 Horacio Fabrega, Jr., 'Medical anthropology', in B. J. Siegal (ed.), *Biennial Review of Anthropology,* Stanford, California, Stanford University Press, 1972, p. 189.

95 Alan Harwood, *Witchcraft, Sorcery, and Social Categories Among The Safwa,* London, Oxford University Press, 1970, p. 77.

Richard W. Lieban

5

Sex Differences and Cultural Dimensions of Medical Phenomena in a Philippine Setting [1]

Introduction

Organic differences between the sexes combined with associated social role distinctions make contrasts in illness and responses to illness between males and females particularly interesting problems for investigating the interplay between biological and cultural influences on medical phenonema.

Females have a longer life expectancy than males, and indications are that biological factors are significantly involved in contrastive mortality rates between the sexes.[2] Women constitutionally seem to have greater resistance to both infectious and degenerative disease.[3] One example of a study that implicates inherent biological factors in differing life expectancies of males and females is that of Madigan who found that mortality rates between monks and nuns, whose similarity in lifestyles minimized sex-role influences on health, were comparable to differences in mortality rates between males and females in the population at large.[4]

While women have lower mortality rates than men, the patterns with regard to morbidity are quite different. Various data from the United States and Great Britain indicate that women there have higher morbidity rates than men and, according to the US data, these morbidity differences cannot be solely accounted for by conditions related to reproduction.[5] Difficulties arise in trying to explain these higher female morbidity rates on the basis of biological differences between the sexes, considering the apparently greater female resistance to infectious and degenerative disease, mentioned above. There is also relevant evidence with regard to psychiatric illnesses. Gove found that while married women in the United States have higher rates of psychiatric illness than married men, such differences do not appear when single, divorced or widowed women are compared with their male counterparts, and he argues that this contradicts the hypothesis that women are biologically more susceptible to such illnesses than men are.[6] While biologically orientated explanations of higher morbidity in women have old roots in medical literature, more recent interpretations have tended to concentrate on social rather than biological stresses of women's roles.[7]

Sex differences are associated with significant differences in reliance on medical systems. More utilization of medical resources by women than men is characteristic in Western medical settings.[8] In non-Western areas, variable patterns have been reported. For example, Press found in Bogota that more women than men utilized both a traditional healer and modern medical resources, with the proportion of women higher in the first instance.[9] On the other hand, Leighton *et al.* found that among the Yoruba of Nigeria more men than women used modern medical facilities, but more women than men relied on traditional healers.[10]

According to data which I collected during a study of traditional medicine in Cebu City, Philippines, twice as many females as males used the services of three of the most popular healers in the city, a ratio, incidentally, unaffected by whether the practitioner was a man or a woman. The ratio of females to males was significantly higher for patients of these traditional healers than for patients of physicians for whom I have data. (The physicians, one a general practitioner and the other an opthamologist, had in several cases treated informants who also had been treated by a healer for the same illness. In random samples of these physicians' records, 56 and 53 per cent of their patients respectively were female.)

If women utilize medical services in a society more frequently than men do, it may be because of higher morbidity rates among women, or – differences in morbidity aside – their greater readiness to seek medical aid, or a combination of both factors. In this chapter, it is the third possibility, as it is affected by culturally defined role differences between men and women in Philippine society, that I would like to explore. In addition, I want to consider possible therapeutic aspects of the traditional medical system in relation to the differential use of healers by men and women in Cebu City. But first, in order to see the argument in perspective, it is necessary to provide some background on the setting and medical context.

Cebu City and Its Medical Resources

Cebu City has the largest urban population of any city in the Philippines outside metropolitan Manila, with a population of more than 340,000.[11] The city is part of the Cebuano-speaking area of the central and southern Philippines, and Cebuanos are one of the major Christian ethnolinguistic groups that constitute more than 85 per cent of the Philippine population. More than 90 per cent of Cebu City's population is Catholic. The city is the capital of Cebu province, and it is a major transportation, trade and manufacturing centre, as well as the location of the most important concentration of educational facilities in the Philippines outside the Manila area. Cebu City is also a medical centre.

At the time I did research in the city, there were more than 150 physicians, 100 pharmacies, and numerous hospitals, major clinics, and X-ray and clinical laboratories. But if the city is a major modern medical centre, it is a centre of traditional medicine as well. Its healers have a substantial following among the city's population, and these healers, especially the most popular and successful of them, attract large numbers of patients from other areas.

Although healers draw most of their patients from the poorer and less educated of the population, many middle- to upper-class individuals rely at times on the help of healers. A dualistic pattern of the utilization of medical services predominates in the city, with greater or less reliance on healers and physicians corresponding respectively to lower and higher positions in the class structure.

In Cebu City and other Cebuano areas there are three principal medical roles. A therapist may specialize in only one, or he may combine two or all of them in his practice. The *mananabang* is the traditional midwife. The *manghihilot,* a masseur or masseuse, is primarily a specialist for treating ailments of the skeletal and muscle systems. The *mananambal* is a general practitioner whose medical role has the greatest scope of any in the traditional system, both in terms of numbers of patients and of variety of illness treated. The three Cebu City healers referred to earlier were *mananambal*, and since it is patients of this type of healer that concern us, discussion of the traditional medical system will concentrate on *mananambal* at this point.

Mananambal have a special connection with the spiritual world which validates their qualification for the role and is the source of their healing power. Most often a *mananambal* first establishes a relationship with the spiritual world in dreams or visions. The spiritual aid the healer claims may come directly from God, Christ, the Virgin Mary, a saint, the spirit of a deceased *mananambal*, or even from deceased national heroes. Usually the ties are with a single spiritual benefactor, but some *mananambal* have more than one source of spiritual support.

Illnesses treated by *mananambal* can be broadly classified into those which (1) have etiologies that are morally neutral: events, conditions and processes of the everyday world; and (2) have causes that reflect a motivated universe, represented by those who have extraordinary powers that can generate illness. The former 'natural' etiologies recognize such causes as irregular habits, exposure to wind or sudden temperature changes, fatigue, faulty diet, emotional states and relapses. The latter 'supernatural' etiologies ascribe causes to sorcery, witchcraft, neglected or possessive ancestral spirits, other spirits outside the pale of God, and God, who may punish certain moral transgressions by sending sickness.

Symptoms of patients and their medical and social histories are important diagnostic cues for *mananambal*. Frequently healers are said to derive from their spiritual benefactors knowledge of their patients' conditions.

To treat illnesses, *mananambal* may employ a variety of remedies, including plants, some of whose healing properties have been noted by physicians[12] and are part of a comprehensive inventory of useful medicinal plants used in the Philippines;[13] certain mechanical and chemical procedures that are of established value and are found in many medical systems, such as massage, cupping, anointing, poulticing and steam inhalations; and various magico-religious therapies, including prayers, incantations and gestures. It should be noted that the *materia medica* and the mechanical and chemical procedures are integrated into a sacred context. In other words, as they are characteristically employed by *mananambal,* an association rather than a contrast between 'material' and 'spiritual' resources is emphasized.

In contrast to physicians, at least those in private practice who see their patients behind closed doors, *mananambal* diagnose and treat their patients in the open, in a much more public fashion. So far as the more popular *mananambal* are concerned, from an outsider's perspective the healer and the patient under treatment can be seen as actors in a kind of 'medicodrama', with an audience of waiting patients, some of whom on occasion may become actors themselves, even before they are treated, when they are asked by the *mananambal* to confirm some indication of his healing power, or they volunteer such information.

The role of the *mananambal* is defined as one of service, and the *mananambal* is not supposed to profit from his healing power. At the same time, the patient is obligated to offer at least some token of gratitude, and in a metropolis such as Cebu City, costs of medical care by some leading *mananambal* may be as high as, or higher than, those incurred under treatment by physicians.

Sex Roles and Stress-Related Morbidity

Having briefly described certain salient features of the medical context in Cebu City, particularly the traditional healing system, we now turn to a basic problem addressed by this paper: how certain sex role differences may help explain the higher proportion of females among patients of *mananambal.* It should be stressed that the factors to be discussed are not intended to account for all of the disproportion, but they may contribute to it. We begin with consideration of differences in normative expectations of behaviour pertaining to men and women that could lead to a higher risk for the latter of morbidity related to certain kinds of stress.

Philippine women are not subject to status deprivation such as that described by Lewis[14] for pastoral Somali women, whose domination by men is seen by him as related to the higher frequency among women of spirit possession, regarded in the culture as an illness and accompanied by parallel symptoms. In contrast, equivalent rights of the sexes, both in the household and the social world outside, is a strong motif of culture in the Philippines.[15] The

following quotation from a housewife in a rural Philippine community may be somewhat extreme in its assertiveness, but it does
reflect a tradition in which women have a strong standing in the
society. The woman in this case is discussing how she gets her husband to co-operate in doing household chores:

> I make him do it most of the time because he is my husband. I
> have to get him to do it for no one will do it for us. I don't want
> him to be the one telling me things. I am the woman.[16]

While in general Philippine wives have rights equivalent to
those of husbands, this parity does not prevail in one aspect of
marital relations. A double standard of constraints on sexual behaviour of males and females begins at the time of courtship in
Christian Filipino society and extends into marriage. In the
family, the importance of modesty and chastity in a daughter is
emphasized, fickle behaviour with young men is generally dis-
approved of, and the family has a strong obligation to protect its
daughter's virtue before marriage. In contrast, society is far more
permissive when it comes to premarital sexual experiences of
young men, and success in this regard is an important source of
prestige for bachelors.[17] In marriage, the stability and fidelity of
the wife are stressed, and she is expected to be the rock of the
family; husbands are not subject to comparable pressures to
behave as responsibly.[18]

The influence of this normative double standard on actual behaviour can be seen in sorcery cases, which are reflections of social
strains. In sorcery cases which I collected that involved residents
of Cebu City, the largest number was attributed by informants to
antagonisms connected with courtship or marriage.[19] With the
differences in behavioural orientation between males and females
before marriage, it might be expected that when sorcery cases are
thought to be related to the ending of a romance at the initiative
of one of the parties, in most instances the one to withdraw from
the relationship would be the young man rather than the young
woman. This was the situation in nine of the thirteen cases of this
kind on which I have data. Considering marriage, in instances
where marital infidelity is believed to be the cause of conflict that
precipitates a sorcery attack, the number of cases in which husbands rather than wives were unfaithful could be expected to be

greater, considering the stronger constraints on wives with respect to violation of marital vows. And in six of the seven cases on which I have data that involve marital infidelity, the husband was the transgressor.

The greater likelihood that when infidelity occurs in marriage, it will be the husband rather than the wife who is unfaithful is reflected in other data. One *mananambal* who was my informant not only treated patients but also offered help to people who came to her with other problems. For many of those who sought her assistance, the problem was the infidelity of a spouse. Assistance would be requested from the spiritual benefactor of the *mananambal* in such ways as asking him to help the wayward spouse to return to the fold of the family, or punishing the mistress of the husband until she gave him up. I obtained data on sixty such cases, and in all but five the individual complaining about the infidelity of a spouse was the wife.[20]

It is one thing to have evidence that more wives than husbands are subject to stress connected with suspicion or knowledge of marital infidelity of a spouse. It is quite another matter to establish that such stress can be related to symptoms of illness that might send an affected individual to a healer for medical help. Data from a study by a Manila psychiatrist are helpful in this regard. Lapuz, the psychiatrist, made a study of a sample of her patients with a variety of psychiatric ailments other than psychoses. Among married women in her sample, the most grievous fault of a husband was considered to be his involvement with another woman, and discovery of such involvement 'provoked a major emotional upheaval, with hysterical outbursts, a deluge of somatic ailments and seemingly endless self-torturing obsessions about the traumatic event'.[21]

Data such as these indicate that the double standard of sexual behaviour can have epidemiological as well as social significance, and cases of this kind demonstrate that illness can be a consequence of social as well as biological processes.

The fact that under such circumstances stress can be conducive to somatic symptomatology also has a bearing on the greater utilization of *mananambal* by women than men. This is so because in virtually all cases where I observed *mananambal* treat a patient, the patient complained of organic symptoms. Therefore, in cases where marital stresses of the kind we have been considering are related to symptoms of the patient, women, who outnumber men in being subject to these stresses, would outnumber them as patients.

Sex Differences and the Recognition of Illness

So far we have considered how sex-role differences can be assotiated with higher rates of morbidity for Philippine women. Now we want to consider how, differences in morbidity aside, cultural expectations of their society may make Philippine women in the Cebuano area readier than men to define themselves as ill and in need of medical treatment.

The idea that women are more susceptible to illness than men is expressed in the etiology of Cebuano traditional medicine. The traditional disease concept *bughat,* which has a variety of meanings, is crucial in this respect.

Bughat is a general designation for relapse. Factors which *mananambal* said can bring about a relapse include physical stresses, such as overwork or taking a rough bus trip; taking a bath too soon after remission of symptoms; eating too much or too little and missing meals at regular times; anger and, particularly, eating the wrong foods during or shortly after recovery. Examples of diet items proscribed by one *mananambal* because they could cause a relapse were: (1) 'Bloody' fish, which can have an adverse effect on a person who is recovering from 'an illness, although not on someone who is well. (2) Cuttle fish – because it 'looks like a tumour', and when sick 'it is not good to eat a disease'. (3) Carabao and chicken – because they are 'hot'. (The last statement reflects notions about hot and cold diseases, medicines and foods that are widespread among Filipinos and may be based on ideas derived from Hippocratic medical theory of body humours and pathology and brought to the Philippines by Spanish colonizers.)[22]

In addition to its general meaning of relapse, the term *bughat* also refers to specific female ailments, and it is these aspects of the term that especially interest us. The ailments in question, as they are classified in the traditional medical system, are all related to the female reproductive system.

One class of *bughat* ailments pertains to menstrual irregularities. In women who have not had a child, the principal cause of this is said to be deviation from the rule that one should not take a bath within eight days after menstruation begins. Other causes are overwork or exposure to too much heat, from the sun or a stove, which can 'thicken the blood'. Women who have had children can also have menstrual problems precipitated by these factors and, in addition, complications from parturition are thought to be a major cause of subsequent menstrual difficulties. According to traditional medical theory, a woman should bleed for approximately one month after parturition, and if she does not, the 'bad blood', which should be discharged, accumulates in the body causing menstrual irregularities and possible associate symptoms, such as swollen abdomen, headaches, and, in some cases, fever.

When it comes to menstrual problems, difficulties experienced by women who have not had a child are distinguished from those of women who have had a child as different kinds of *bughat* and treated differently even when the condition is immediately pre-cipitated by the same factor (such as premature bathing in rela-tion to the menstrual cycle). This reflects the fact that parturition is thought to make women who have experienced it vulnerable to illness in a special way that is not shared with females who have not had a child, and this vulnerability is an essential part of the etiology when the former develop a variety of ailments. Except for menstrual difficulties, all other uses of the term *bughat* to designate female sicknesses refer to maladies of women with this special vul-nerability, a vulnerability that begins with the puerperium.

Various measures are taken to safeguard the health of the mother and prevent a relapse after parturition. These include rest and special diet. 'Mother roasting', a widespread traditional practice in Southeast Asia, is part of the puerperium regimen in various areas of the Philippines, Christian[23] as well as 'tribal',[24] although it is by no means found throughout the archipelago to-day.[25] To give some idea of the importance that prophylaxis during the puerperium can assume for one Philippine group, the Subanun of Mindanao, Frake and Frake contrast the Subanun view of the dangerous part of the reproductive experience with that in Western society.

Modern medical practice prescribes only a variable period of rest as essential for normal post-natal patients. . . . The major attention of the physician and the concern of the patient are

directed to the delivery itself and to pregnancy. Once a successful birth has occurred, elation replaces anxiety. . . .

Among the Subanun, in contrast, a successful birth initiates
a time of fear and concern. They consider the post-natal period
to be critical for the health of the mother and infant. Following
delivery, Subanun culture prescribes not celebration but a
course of intensive medical care.[26]

While the puerperium is regarded as a time of risk for the
mother in Cebuano areas of the Philippines, the childbirth experience is thought to make the mother vulnerable to *bughat* far
beyond the puerperium. I have heard a woman's illness diagnosed
as *bughat* when her last child had been born more than thirty
years before. As *mananambal* explain it, the birth of a child
stretches the muscles of the mother – two used the metaphor of
'loosening the nuts and bolts of the woman's body' – lowering her
resistance to illness for the rest of her life. Following are some
examples of cases diagnosed as *bughat* in which the persisting
effect of parturition beyond the puerperium makes the patient's
body vulnerable to an insult that precipitates the illness.

A woman has just come in to be treated by the *mananambal,*
and she complains of pain in one shoulder and fatigue. The
patient had her last child more than twenty years before. She
diagnoses her ailment as *bughat* due to overwork, slicing and
pounding banana stalks for pigs, and the *mananambal* agrees
with her diagnosis.

In another case, a *mananambal* has diagnosed his patient's
illness as *bughat* brought on by overwork. The woman has
children, although none newborn, and the healer states that she
asks her children to help with household chores and they will
not, so she does everything herself. The healer goes on to say
that this is what happens when parents spoil their children.

A third case is that of a woman who has come to a *mananambal* with a severe headache. The healer moves her lips in silent
prayer while massaging her patient's forehead with oil. After
several minutes of treatment, the patient appears to be much
improved, and when she leaves she says she knows how to smile
again. The *mananambal* says this is a case of *bughat* due to
constant worry by the patient about her ability to support her
children since the death of her husband two years before.

Another case involves a woman who complains that her eyes

are tired and they feel as if they have particles of sand in them. The healer diagnoses this as *bughat* due to the combination of a lack of sleep and too much sorrow, the *mananambal* explaining that the woman had been swindled out of a large amount of money two years before.

As a general term for relapse, *bughat* refers to a recurrence of symptoms of an illness which had abated, and in this sense it is similar to the meaning of the word 'relapse' in English. The relapse is a renewal of the original illness. But the term *bughat* as used in the above four cases can denote sickness that bears no relationship to an illness in the past. Perhaps an underlying link between the general meaning of *bughat* as relapse and its special application to ailments of women who have had children is that illness in each is related to a prior trauma that makes the body more susceptible to subsequent morbidity. Once a woman has given birth to a child, this special susceptibility is lifelong.

In *bughat* cases of this kind, the vulnerability of the woman is a constant in the etiology; the factors which can precipitate the illness are variable. They are primarily emotional, or have such connotations, and include anger, worry, excitement, shock, overwork, grief, shouting, improper or irregular diet, and lack of sleep. Symptoms of cases observed include headache, fever, pain, numbness, fatigue, uneasiness, diarrhoea, nausea, lesions, swelling, weakness, and difficulty in breathing.

The *bughat* etiology suggests that perhaps more women than men assume the sick role at least in part because women are more inclined to interpret certain disvalued sensations and conditions as illness, related to the greater cultural licence they have to be sick. This could help explain why *mananambal* have more female than male patients.

In exploring a way in which culture can be involved in the subjective aspects of certain illnesses, there is no intention to disregard the importance of morbidity of patients of *mananambal*. Many patients of healers, both men and women, who were observed, had serious organic dysfunctions. But evaluation of possible signs of illness by the individual who has them and others who influence him is an essential part of the process by which the individual decides he is sick.[27] And in instances where the signs are minor or ambiguous, an etiology that says women are more susceptible to illness than men are is likely to 'create' more sick women than men.

Under the circumstances, it could be expected that proportionately more female than male patients will come to the *mananambal* with secondary ailments, and considering the importance of emotional factors in the traditional etiology of *bughat*, it seems likely that psychosomatic factors are implicated in many *bughat* cases. Implications of this in relation to therapeutic resources offered by *mananambal* will be considered next.

Illnesses, Sex Differences and the Healer's Therapy

Thus far, we have discussed how cultural norms associated with sex differences may in certain respects produce higher rates of morbidity and regardless of morbidity, higher rates of perceived illness among Cebuano women than men. I would like to consider whether characteristics of illnesses of the kind we have been discussing may make many of these illnesses conducive to favourable responses of patients to treatment by the healer.

As we have seen, certain marital stresses to which women are especially subject can be related to somatic symptoms, and the prominence of emotional factors in the etiology of *bughat* suggests that there may be an important psychosomatic component in many cases diagnosed as *bughat*. Under these circumstances, numerous illnesses of the kind we have been considering could be responsive to psychotherapy.

In a recent paper,[28] I tried to analyse why the most popular *mananambal* in Cebu City, such as the three healers whose practices are discussed in the present paper, have so many more patients than some of their less illustrious counterparts. An important difference between healers lies in the signification of their healing power. Through their behaviour, the most popular *mananambal* frequently indicate the presence and help of their spiritual patrons when treating patients. This is much less true of less popular healers who usually have had at least one or a series of mystical experiences that signify some special calling or connection with the spiritual world, but who do not characteristically behave during treatment in ways that indicate the actual presence and aid of a spiritual source of healing power. In addition, patients of the less popular healers are exposed to far fewer indications of the healers' accomplishments than patients of the leading *mananambal*. This is true not only because the leading *mananambal* more often assert their success, but also because their patients are much more likely to be in the company of other patients waiting for treatment, and in situations where the most popular *mananambal* practise, their claims are often augmented by testimonials from their patients.

Mananambal in Cebu City generally rely less on *materia medica* than rural healers do, and more and less popular healers of the city do not seem to differ significantly in this respect. Under these circumstances, the best medicine of the *mananambal* could be the patient's impression of his healing power, and the most popular healers, who foster the strongest impression of conveying that power, may also be the most effective. This is a proposition that is consistent with psychiatric interpretations such as that of Frank[29] who emphasizes the importance of persuasion in healing, and sees an arousal of hope in the patient, associated with his dependence on the healer, as central to the effectiveness of religious and magical therapy.[30]

Frank[31] distinguishes two types of consequences of psycho-therapy: symptom relief, which is rapid and primarily depends on the expectations of help, and improved functioning, which depends not only on a learning process that is accelerated by the therapist but also on social interactions outside the therapeutic relationship. For the most part, contact of *mananambal* with patients are brief, focused on the immediate medical problem of the patient, and not concerned with developing the patient's insight or with social intervention on his behalf. Given these characteristics of healing style, it seems likely that the psychotherapeutic potential of the *mananambal*'s treatment would be for the relief of symptoms. Pertinent in this connection are findings of a psychiatrist, Shakman,[32] who interviewed twenty-three healers in various parts of the Philippines, questioned seventy-four of their patients and observed treatment of patients. He presents case materials on five of these patients, all women with somatic complaints, whom he regarded as suffering from psychogenic disorders and who responded favourably to treatment in the healing setting. On the basis of his observations, Shakman[33] stated that the 'most impressively supernatural rituals are most effective'.

Conclusion

In this chapter, we began with a basic biological distinction between men and women, and have considered how cultural factors associated with these organic differences may influence illness and responses to treatment of illness. In so doing, our intention has not been to slight the significance of biological dimensions of medicine, but in bringing a social science perspective to certain problems, our emphasis has been on social, cultural and behavioural aspects of illness and its treatment.

Modern medicine has had an intensive biomedical focus, which has been the source of impressive accomplishments, but also the source of limitations. And various observers have suggested the need to develop new or modified paradigms of medical knowledge that will give adequate recognition to medical ramifications of social, cultural and behavioural factors.[34]

Such ramifications have been the subject of this chapter which has explored how certain beliefs and related behaviour may influence the differential utilization of Cebuano healers by men and women. The beliefs in question concern marital obligations of husbands and wives, differences in body image pertaining to men and women and the spiritual basis of healing. These beliefs are part of Cebuano basic domains of thought concerning the nature of man, society and the cosmos. In this perspective, we have been considering how medical phenomena may be shaped by the ontology of a society as well as by biological factors.

NOTES AND REFERENCES

1   Field research for this study was supported by a grant from the National Science Foundation.

2   D. Mechanic, *Medical Sociology,* New York, Free Press, 1968.

3   C. A. Natanson, 'Illness and the feminine role: a theoretical review', *Social Science and Medicine,* Vol. 9, 1975, pp. 57-62.

4   F. C. Madigan, 'Are sex morbidity differentials biologically caused?', *Milbank Memorial Quarterly,* Vol. 35, 1957, pp. 202-23.

5   C. A. Natanson, op. cit.

6   W. Gove, 'The relationship between sex roles, marital status and mental illness', *Social Forces,* Vol. 51, 1972, pp. 34-53.

7   C. A. Natanson, op. cit.

8   See O. W. Anderson, 'The utilization of health services', in H. Freeman, S. Levine and L. G. Reeder (eds.), *Handbook of Medical Sociology,* Englewood Cliffs, Prentice Hall, 1963, pp. 349-68.

9   I. Press, 'Urban illness: physicians, curers and dual use in Bogota', *Journal of Health and Social Behaviour,* Vol. 10, 1969, pp. 209-18.

10   A. H. Leighton, *et al., Psychiatric Disorder among the Yoruba,* Ithaca, Cornell Universiy Press, 1963.

11   *Cebu Census of Population and Housing,* Manila, Bureau of the Census and Statistics, 1972.

12   R. Lieban, *Cebuano Sorcery: Malign Magic in the Philippines,* Berkeley and Los Angeles, University of California Press, 1967.

13   E. Quisumbing, *Medicinal plants of the Philippines,* Republic of the Philippines Department of Agriculture and Natural Resources, Technical Bulletin No. 16, Manila, Republic of the Philippines Bureau of Printing, 1951.

14   I. M. Lewis, *Ecstatic Religion: an Anthropological Study of Spirit Possession and Shamanism,* Harmondsworth, Penguin Books, 1971.

15   See G. M. Guthine, *The Filipino child and Philippine society,* Manila, Philippine Normal College Press, 1961; R. B. Fox, 'Men and women in the Philippines', in B. E. Ward (ed.), *Women in the New Asia,* Paris, UNESCO, 1963.

16   E. Nurge, *Life in a Leyte village,* Seattle, University of Washington Press, 1965.

17   A. P. Pal, 'A Philippine barrio', *University of Manila Journal of East Asiatic Studies,* Vol. 5, 1956, p. 333.

18   J. Bulatao, 'Philippine values I: the Manileno's mainsprings', *Philippine Studies,* Vol. 10, 1962, pp. 54-67.

19   R. Lieban, op. cit.

20   R. Lieban, 'Shamanism and social control in a Philippine city', *Journal of the Folklore Institute,* Vol. 11, 1965, pp. 43-54.

21   L. V. Lapuz, *A Study of Psychopathology,* Quezon City, University of the Philippines Press, 1973.

22   In this connection, see D. V. Hart, *Bisayan Filipino and Malayan Humoral Pathologies: Folk Medicine and Ethno-history in Southeast Asia,* Southeast Asian Program, Data Paper No. 76, Ithaca, Deparment of Asian Studies, Cornell University, 1969.

23   See W. F. Nydegger and C. Nydegger, *Tarong: an Ilocos Barrio in the Philippines,* New York, London and Sydney, John Wiley, 1966; F. L. Jocano, *Folk Medicine in a Philippine Municipality,* Manila, The National Museum, 1973.

24 C. O. Frake and C. M. Frake, 'Post-natal care among the Eastern Subanun', *The Silliman Journal*, Vol. 4, 1957, pp. 207-15.

25 D. V. Hart, 'From pregnancy through birth in a Bisayan Filipino village', in D. V. Hart *et al., Southeast Asian Birth Customs: Three Studies in Human Reproduction,* New Haven, Human Relations Area Files Press, 1965.

26 C. O. Frake and C. M. Frake, op. cit.

27 Organic criteria tend to dominate our concept of illness. Certainly this has been so from the perspective of modern medicine, which has concentrated much of its attention on the organism and disease processes. Yet even in modern industrial societies a strictly organic concept of illness begins to founder in the face of evidence such as that which shows that many people who are professionally diagnosed as having something organically wrong with them don't regard themselves as ill, and many who go to physicians demonstrate no definable pathology. In other words, for patients and non-patients, illness has a subjective meaning that may not correspond to organic pathology as defined by biomedical science. See J. R. Audi, 'Measurement and diagnosis of health', in P. Shepherd and D. McKinley (eds.), *Environmental Essays on the Planet as Home,* Boston, Houghton-Mifflin, 1971; H. P. Dreitzel, 'Introduction', in H. P. Dreitzel (ed.), *The Social Organization of Health,* New York, Macmillan, 1971.

28 R. Lieban, 'Symbols, signs, and success: healers and power in a Philippine city', in R. D. Fogelson and R. Adams (eds.), *The Anthropology of Power,* New York, Academic Press, 1977, pp. 57-66.

29 J. Frank, *Persuasion and Healing,* Baltimore, The Johns Hopkins University Press, 1961.

30 A. Kiev, *Transcultural Psychiatry,* New York, Free Press, 1972.

31 J. Frank, op. cit.

32 R. Shakman, 'Indigenous healing of mental illness in the Philippines', *The International Journal of Social Psychiatry,* Vol. 15, 1969, pp. 279-87.

33 Ibid., p. 285.

34 See I. Galdston, 'Retrospect and prospect', in I. Galdston (ed.), *Man's Image in Medicine and Anthropology,* New York, International Universities Press, 1963; J. Cassel, 'Social science theory as a source of hypotheses in epidemiological research', *American Journal of Public Health*, Vol. 54, 1964, pp. 1482-8; H. Fabrega, 'The need for an ethnomedical science', *Science,* Vol. 189, 1975, pp. 969-75.

Lola Romanucci-Ross

6

Melanesian Medicine: Beyond Culture to Method

The body of materials gathered on sickness and health, healing and curing rites has reached a magnitude that pre-empts further collection without insistence on a 'frame' for the sets of domains which will allow comparison and contrast. Medical systems elicited by investigators from many diverse cultures can now be looked at for points of congruence and divergence along the similarity-difference continuum. This requires operational frames of great flexibility which permit the viewing of thought systems in the recognition that there are knowledge configurations, not just a body of knowledge.

To go beyond culture is to begin to understand that we have confused magnitude with complexity, and in our reductionistic preoccupation with analysis, in medical anthropology, we have neglected to relate medical events to the totality of systems in the culture we are studying. Through our method of participant observation we have neglected participatory understanding. Ethnoscience, viewing the world through the categories of other cultures, encourages a consciousness of method in cultural investigation. Like cultural relativism it provides insights; but it also creates serious problems. For the cultural relativist, the 'good' is defined only in its total cultural context. Is there, then, no absolute, ultimate good? For the ethnoscientist, knowledge is always relative to cultural categorization. Is there, then, no ultimate reality? My purpose in this chapter is to indicate, through a consideration of Melanesian medicine, that in event-structure analysis the commonality of cross-cultural experience can allow us to transcend the differences between the categories of the investigating culture and the informing culture to achieve further understanding.

My approach here will be to expose an analytic mode encompassing body-mind as a unit firmly articulated in personhood in a hierarchy of systems and to view those intersects which subject the entire system to stress, as well as processes invoked or employed to restore system balance. This modelic will reference, in particular, two villages of the Matankor peoples of the Admiralty Islands, inhabited by the Sori and the Mokerang. The Sori, who will receive the greater emphasis, were relatively isolated at the time of my fieldwork,[1] whereas the Mokerang had a history 'from the time of the Germans' of persistent, if not intense, contact with European culture.[2]

The narrative may appear to 'need sorting' into what we construe as varied and separate realities: myth, history, kinship, navigation, medical clinical trials, and medical research strategies, professional training, neolithic sciences, but it stands written in the Matankor *mode* as part of *their* philosophy of science to the extent that I was able to perceive it and translate it to my comprehension. If 'I' appear in the setting, it is because I, and not someone else, was there; it is an attempt to be more, not less, objective.

Illness, not music, is the universal language. This heretical notion came to light in Melanesia during the morning medical line-up, as I played doctor-patient rather than anthropologist-informant with the villagers. The evening musicals around my record player registered the fact that my Sori friends didn't 'hear' Mozart, just as the flute players of the Sepik did not respond to European flute virtuosity.

But shared fear of body-mind breakdown made instant intimates of strangers. This was further demonstrated in Los Angeles, as my Mexican friend Amparo met with John Kilepak Kisokau, our former Manus boat crew captain. Amparo and John began to communicate through my neo-Melanesian and Mexican-Spanish translations as he nourished hopes for her favour and she satisfied her curiosity about a pierced-eared and tattooed 'savage'. The initial total alienation ('Ask him if he was born with those huge holes in his earlobes') evolved to empathy ('Tell her these tattoo marks were for the bloodletting that cured my severe headaches'). The rest of the morning was filled with fast and informative queries and responses on how to substitute materials available in

Los Angeles for obsidian, and which magical medicine would cure her father of his witchcraft-induced alcoholism. Amparo told John of strange cures in Mexico. He wanted to be very sure that she understood that perhaps some of his cures worked only in the Admiralties and certainly only if the proper kin was involved. In their shared anxieties and excitement over remedies, categories of 'folk' and 'primitive' dissolved for this observer.

If we are to understand illness as the universal language, we may begin by looking further into the analytical mode of the Melanesian.

The Admiralty Islands

Situated about 150 miles north of New Guinea, the Admiralties constitute a small archipelago at 2°S latitude, and 147°E longitude. The Admiralty group consists of the main high island of Manus and about fifteen smaller outliers of the mixed volcanic and coral types. Manus is about fifty miles long and twenty miles wide; it is largely mountainous, peaking at 3,000 feet. The population consists of about 20,000 natives from approximately twenty linguistic groups, as recognized by them. A huge naval base was built on Manus during World War II, and it was one of the arenas of actual combat. A few hundred 'Europeans' (mainly Australians) and some Chinese lived in the administrative town of Lorengau or at the nearby naval base at Lombrum. Mokerang village is a few miles from the naval base, while Saapoy is quite isolated on the north coast, requiring a long canoe trip of perhaps two days in the absence of the north-west monsoons (during these times one doesn't get in or out of Sori territory).

Admiralty Islanders classify themselves into three groups. The sea-going Manus live by fishing and trade, domiciled in pile-house villages over shallow lagoons between fringing reefs and the shore; since 1948 they have lived on the beach, however. The Matankor, such as the Sori and Mokerang, live on small islands around the Great Admiralty (Manus), and combine fishing with gardening and tree crop cultivation. The Usiai people of the interior of Manus, the 'bush people', are gardeners exclusively. The Bismarck Archipelago and New Guinea were administered by Germany from 1884 to 1914 with the Australians assuming control in World

War I. From the 1880s to the present, some of the natives, particularly those of the south coast, have served in European employ working on ships or plantations or in towns. Contacts with Christian missions began in German times, continued under the Australian Administration, and some (Catholic, Lutheran, Seventh Day Adventists) were established with permanence. The United Nations placed the area under Australia as a Trust Territory in 1946; internal self-government was instituted in 1973 and full independence in 1975.

Previous Studies – An Introduction to Discourse on Method

To anthropologists of the past, remote and recent, anyone's illness was a nuisance to the field investigator. Medicine-magic-religion came as a package in shaman-observed studies, and we still go about untangling the threads of this trinity. Ethnosemantics resolved many of the seeming paradoxes.[3]

The present status of medical anthropology is described in a rather complete exposition by Horacio Fabrega.[4] The ethnomedical approach, in which illness is viewed according to internally defined cultural categories, has been used by anthropologists in many parts of the 'primitive', 'peasant', and 'underdeveloped' world. Studies have focused on sorcery, folk psychiatry, the historical contingency of culture contact situations, religious beliefs and curing. There have been descriptions and analyses of folk illness with attempts to link these to socio-psychological change and stress; there have been studies on 'possession' behaviour and on the family's reaction to such behaviour. Native categories of illness have been described.

I had noticed that my field notes in Mexico were replete with references to illnesses, and that, indeed, illness was the lynchpin of much village discourse and much that occurred in the village.[5] Illness was the opener to many a conversation and often the dramatic climax in conflict situations, major and minor. Yet with professional *disinvoltura* I went to Melanesia disjoined from this awareness. An Australian physician in New Britain drew my attention to the cultural aspects of illness because of his need as a physician to be more effective as such in the territories. Using the statistical and descriptive material which I had collected in my own fieldwork and that available from the field notes of Theodore Schwartz, Reo Fortune and Margaret Mead, I wrote about shifting 'game' strategies in curing events, when the choices were many and reflected varying degrees of deculturation and acculturation.[6] Priorities and sequentiality of selected curing procedures could be predicted. Disease causes were distinguishable through several categories: impersonal or interpersonal, the latter further discriminated by soul damage caused by cursing within the group, or sorcery outside of the group. Supra-human agents of disease could be outside the body or immanent. Natives credited Western medicine with excellent descriptive categories and precise instrumentation but judged it poor in explanatory models: 'What good is your medicine if you can't tell me why I got sick?'

Because the somatic drama is culturally informed, it seems not inappropriate to consider the illness-health continuum as grounded in sensory perceptions of the world, and the manner in which these are registered as knowledge-configurations which provide the guide for further perceiving. Culturally informed imagery not only includes, but possibly begins with, and is derivative of, proprioception: 'body image' in space and time affected by group processes. How is consensus arrived at from the syntactical to the rhetorical and from the 'coding' on many levels of the organization of experience? How are the rules for articulation of levels arrived at? Some homely examples of lack of awareness of such considerations follow.

The Costly Experiment of Ad Hoc Solutions to Public Health Problems in Culture-Contact Situations

Because of continuing contact with Europeans, a New Guinean now has a life expectancy of about sixty years. Infant mortality has dropped from between 200 to 400 per thousand to 66 per thousand. The population is now outstripping the food supply and there is widespread malnutrition. Emerging employment patterns indicate that the men are going off to plantations, or to the centres of Lae, Madang, Rabaul. Young people have been going off to high schools and even to colleges in Australia.[7]

With the disintegration of the clan, care for the aged and the reciprocal responsibility between members disappeared. What is referred to as better medical care consists of keeping more people alive longer and allowing more people to be born. The birth rate shows a 7 per cent surplus of births over deaths. In their own family planning scheme of the past, married men slept more nights in the men's house, or on long fishing trips, than they did with their wives; there were many taboos and negative sanctions on intercourse, such as the obligation to pay the husband of the woman in adultery; simultaneous pregnancies among co-wives and years of nursing babies precluded intercourse.

The new woman of New Guinea, however, emulates our sexual availability and has adopted other 'evolved' practices such as bottle feeding (without access to canned baby foods and vitamin supplements). Advanced cultures are there to prepare the New Guineans on all fronts with intra-uterine devices and vasectomies and attempts at the sale of condoms and 'the pill'. Newborn babies, because of better pre-natal care and changing life styles are increasing in weight and size, while pelvic sizes remain the same. Many women now suffer long and difficult labour (24-48 hours), readily incurring infection and peritonitis. (It has been recorded by other investigators, as well as by me, that labour for these women was normally brief, relatively painless, and without incident.) The incidence of venereal disease is rising swiftly, with many previous encumbrances to its spread removed in the rapid culture change.

Some medical researchers feel that the affliction of the swollen-bellied children, *enteritis necroticans* associated with *clostridium perifringens,* type F, is caused by sudden protein infusion into a body which does not have the enzymes to deal with it. This may or may not be true, but the population has adapted to surviving and reproducing on low-protein diets; as a remedy it is now being suggested that they grow peanuts, wheat and maize to hasten the adaptation. The reader is referred to the similar neolithization process of the American Indians, and its unhappy 'public health' consequences, when perfectly adapted hunter-gatherers were turned into farmers.[8]

The low-protein evolutionary adaptation of certain New Guinean tribes may not be our idea of an optimal one. However, once system interference has begun, the interfering culture must be prepared to provide reparations at many points of the contact interface to prevent system disintegration. The 'system', of course, is the people who make up the system and the cost is theirs when the balance is lost.

An undisturbed population, prior to 'conversion', has a knowledge of cultural stochastic process, that is, an ability to predict the sequentiality of events and event probability in alternative hypothetical states.[9] Therefore, the agents of culture change should reach for a level of sophistication comparable to that of their informants.

On Being in the World

Whether we begin with Mantankor exteroception or proprioception, most of the self, if not all of the self, is outside of one. The world is conceived of as flat. From both the Sori and Mokerang I received a description of an earth 'plane' going off in directions, the end points of which would define a circle. Since World War II the circle has become larger and there is more cultural diversity than imagined formerly. In olden times, in one direction were to be found the light-skinned people of 'Yap', and in another the ferocious New Guinea tribesmen with their *sanguman* (evil black magic).

On the Origin of the Human Species

There is nothing irrational to the Mokerang about having the race of man evolve from two drops of blood cultured into fish-hawk and snake before becoming human through various adventures. The blood came from the finger of an old woman who injured herself cleaning clams. The Sori, however, possess an 'island of women' classic, as follows: a group of women on Noru Island had neither husbands nor lovers; the sea gave them pleasure and children. If the newborn was male, it was killed. These women in a *tubweng* (kind of glee) clapped their hands in the ocean and sang '*Arup* (first-born female), *Asang* (second-born female), where are the two men and where is the famous spear called *Nyowena*?' Actually, the spear and the experts were on the mainland hunting in the bush. One day, annoyed by such taunts and the situation in general, these two decided to kill all of the women of Noru. And so they did, not with spearheads of stone or obsidian, but of parinarium nut. All the women were killed except one, who was pregnant. She escaped to big Sori Island and bore a son, who later sired, through her, the founders of the clans Luhai, Hiinang, Saapoy and Babi. Each of these settled a quadrant of the island.

In another myth, a man having eaten bad magic white yams, becomes pregnant; he is horrified by his awareness that he will be unable to give birth. During labour he cuts his belly to deliver himself of twin girls. After wiping them off with seaweed, he expires, having named them *Arup* and *Asap*. They live on seawater for nourishment and then are married by a young man, who examines them first to assure that they are not *marsalai* (bush spirits).

The Totemic Vector

If totemism is an illusion[10] among the Sori, it is an illusion shared by its participants and this investigator. One entered a totemic relationship through the matriline; the original emblem-bearer was a woman who came from Salien to give her female descendants the totem. Salien woman was whisked off to her snake-husband Lapa-Lokoyan by a flying enchanted tree. From his ashes, lovingly cherished by her, there emerged a human being, founder of the Lindrow people, with whom the Sori recognize kinship. The totem given her female descendants would protect their offspring from illness, physical and mental birth defects and body malfunctions, provided the totemic creature was accorded proper respect. Having the *manuay* (fish-hawk) as a totem gave the mother a heavy burden of responsibility for the health of her child. If the *manuay* mother broke any of the taboos (and she could not always know that her 'walkabout' or her canoe had not crossed a spot where a *manuay* had died) her child might never be able to talk, might become paralysed, or at the very least have convulsive seizures with high temperatures. In her right mind, no such mother would risk killing or eating her totemic bird. I was told about the husband of such a woman who took a *manuay* as a pet. He fed it, cared for it, and when it died he buried it. With affection he cut off its foot and put it over the child's pandanus sleeping mat, for protection. The child never learned to talk. The women who told me of this continued by imitating the child's efforts to talk, and editorialized, with horror, that males are often the simple-minded causes of such tragedies. Some men are so careless and stupid when canoeing with their *manuay* wives that barrenness is a common result.

The 'Island of Women' myth seems to be a constant behaviour determinant of male-female relationships. When my five-month-old baby became very ill, I was told that the baby's father probably caused me to offend my totem. I denied having a totemic affiliation. I was told with affectionate impatience that I certainly did have one but simply didn't know what it was! A double jeopardy!

Totemism is a relationship of affect and trust between select humans and select species in which each acts as guardian for the perpetuation of the other. Is there a remedy when this trust is violated? In the event of affliction through broken *manuay* taboos, Tata Tara BwaLohai (widow of Lohai), the oldest woman in the village, is called for curing. The mother of the sick child cooks *saksak* with water and coconut oil. Tata and the other female members of this totemic matriline go to the pandanus-leaf house on piles at an hour when everyone is in the deepest possible slumber. This proper time is reckoned as a segment of time sufficiently in the dead-of-night, but just before dawn. The curing ensemble of women sit in a circle, each with a bit of sago. Tato puts a pandanus-leaf raincape and a *tanket* (croton leaf) over the mother's head. She utters a word not understood by anyone present, herself included, to the *manuay*. The child will be well now. Although there is no signal from the invoked *manuay* to this effect, his warning cry was heard distinctly by the mother before the child became sick.

One man who did not call Tata has three dead children. He insisted that these illnesses were due to bush magic and hence called a *tamberan* from Lebei Village on the mainland. An incredibly naïve diagnosis, according to the women, because his wife is a *manuay* and had broken taboos while pregnant. She had wanted to call Tata but could not go against her husband and that old fool of her father-in-law. Besides these three dead of *manuay* sickness, there were two children of another son of a foolish old man who caught and cooked a *bai-manuay* fish, which was his *uawu* (totem identity) through his mother. The women said, 'Of course, if you ask him "What is your *uawu*?" as you did to us, he will deny that he had one in order to deny his guilt in the death of his grandchildren.'

Can Tata cure anything else? Yes, she has cured barrenness. She has brought back the flow of milk to the breasts of the mother. She 'inoculates' the returned voyager by a cleansing ritual (milk of fresh coconut poured over *tanket* on raincape and words not understood). These had been exposed to soul-stuff pilfering ghosts, bush devils or evil humans who have chewed the leaf with lime and betel nut and spit it out, wishing illness on the stranger in their midst. She can fix broken bones. She is also the keeper of myths and history and astronomical data. Is there anything she cannot cure? Tata replies with laughter 'Yes, Misis, I cannot cure my own knee, and the pain almost kills me.'

Tata's totem is not only the *manuay*. It is also *dyang,* which is the name of a fish, but also means 'sun'. She has a double primary totem, double protection but twice as much risk. The *dyang* taboo applies to both sun and fish. You must not eat either, and in the case of the former this means the sun's rays must not fall upon your cooking utensil. If one ate his *uawu* his teeth would fall out immediately. His skin would fall off. Would he die? No. I can paraphrase what was said to me in this way: one must suffer the consequences in full consciousness of having offended the totem. In the case of Salai (Tata's daughter), neither she nor her new-born baby should be in the sun for one week. If they were, Salai would become very ill, lose her milk, and the baby's skin would be ruined. After the taboo period, the mother of the parturent must take the baby to the sea for bathing. 'Danger is now finished.'

Readers (and some writers) of totemic etiquette may wonder at the apparent foolishness of permanently depriving oneself of a food source as preventive medical insurance. Among these people, being of the *mbu* (banana) totem does not mean you can never eat bananas. An individual has a plurality of totemic relationships; it is possible to have three sets of two combinations. Let us say one can be *mbu/manuay* and *mbu/sa* and *mbu/u* (banana/fish-hawk; banana/bird; banana/cat). You need only take one of these combinations as primary actual. Therefore the *mbu* is not forbidden to you as long as it is duplicated in another set that can negate the first negation in totemic injunction. Pejorative names are also used in this dialectical manner. An epithet can be negated by your giving that name to your brother's daughter. It proves to the world that you have heard the description and reject it. The young lady lives her life for you in total negation of the negation of your existence in another's malevolent consciousness.

The totem can lose its 'strength' or power over its matrilineal membership. Babi, a Mokerang of the crocodile matriline, explained that the eruptions on the scalp of his baby Hibeng had been caused by his handling of three baby crocodiles. The first time he handled them, however, his arm was covered with sores and pustules; the second time nothing happened; and now – Hibeng. His mother Hichepah, however, will still break out in terrible rashes if she handles a baby crocodile.

The young teacher of the elementary school in Mokerang village had 'put it all together now'. His syncretic notion of special creation theory and totemic reality, and the theory of biological evolution was as follows: a long, long time ago, in a time of dreams and mists, God made the world and the animals in it. Certain animals, having evolved from simpler forms, anywhere from six to twelve generations ago, began the matrilines and patrilines of the Admiralty Islands and the New Guinea peoples. Sori, he admitted (as asserted there), was the origin point for matrilineal totems.

The Place

The small island on which the Sori now live was not their original home, Big Sori. (Saapoy Island can be walked, circumferentially, in five minutes, looking out for falling coconuts all the while, and it housed 140 persons during my stay.) The Germans took Big Sori at the turn of this century. They first came to plant coconut trees; a prudent, industrious act which the Sori admired. They were permitted to do so, and those who worked for Germans received small, occasional payments. The Germans then displaced the natives in an act of physical violence, delivering several boxes of *laplap* material and some glass beads to the defeated Sori on the small island. The Sori have heard from some traders that the Germans wrote in a book that the Sori had sold their island. They asked me to write in English that no Sori ever sold their place; one would have had to be crazy to do such a thing for any price, let alone glass beads and *laplaps*!

Saapoy Island is considered split in half, the markers are women's toilet/men's toilet on one side and chief Lohai's house/John Sapalona's canoe on the other. Though the structures are juxtaposed, they belong to different *haps* (halves). The village is further divided into quarters named by wind directions. There are four clans, of mythic origin, each of which contains several patrilines. A deeper existential belonging is to the totemic matriline. Patrilineal membership is used for business, professional and property reasons.

The Sori, placed in a hierarchy of plants and animals, in village segments, genealogical lineages, and totemic memberships, are given role and script for avoidance, marriage, exchange and play relationships. Problem-solving in culture-contact and the *intimate* aspects of male-female relationships are the unprescribed imponderables. The brother-sister pair is nuclear, the source of affection, the locus of exchange not only of fish and sago, but also for the arrangement of a preferred marriage of their children's children, i.e. the children of cross-cousins.

You don't have to marry an actual child of *actual* cross-cousins. A man may say to another from another village, as they work on a plantation, or fish, or meet in a market: 'You are very good to me and from this day forward I shall call you brother.' Thenceforth, all relatives on both sides fall into place as resources for the fictive relation, now actual for practical purposes.

The Making of Babies and Body Image

The Sori despise the Lebei Usiai account of a smoke-eating old man (of dubious human status since he lived with a flying-fox and a bush devil), who was tricked by two desperate women into beginning the art of baby-making. The women disgorged smoke from his belly by spearing him in the anus. Then they fed him cooked food, which is always the first step in assignment of human status. One woman positioned him in the proper topological stance on the other, and as he cried out with need/fear of incontinence, they urged him to 'urinate'. The Sori find this inauspicious beginning of a baby vulgar and idiotic. In their view, they are much more scientific by relying on observation of naturally occurring events. Their observations tell them that a baby 'comes up' as a result of *many* copulatory acts with one or several fathers; existence begins with the co-mingling of male and female fluids in an additive way creating body parts. Resulting parts of the process are fortified and congealed through the menstrual blood which remains in the woman for ten months or a year before 'the face is finished'. Several court cases brought smiles of amusement to village elders who listened to attempts of shamed young women to seek redress: 'So you expect us to believe a baby will be begun after only three times with this man? What do you take us for?'

They did believe that several men sired the newborn, but 'You had better choose one name and stick to it for the Australian court. They believe it is one man, one time, and you won't get anything unless you tell them what they want to hear.'

After marriage, women used to abort by tying a rope tightly around the middle and carrying heavy trees and rocks; although abortion angered the husbands, it was practised under certain circumstances. Other post-marital birth control methods have been indicated earlier.

During labour the belly was rubbed with a leaf called *lawueyeg*; on the south coast the hibiscus flower was similarly used. The female kin gathered, listened to the scream of the young mother that she would die, and subsequently laughed with her that life, not death, had resulted. The deliveries which I was called to assist with did not deviate from this. A baby has a good chance of being well-born if it is full-term and normal. Female helpers do not know how to bring a premature, sickly child into being on their island. They have the important general systems knowledge that their resources cannot support 'life' so defined. Survival on this island is harsh: the *dyapay* monsoon periods cause great hunger. Optimum population is a desideratum always exceeded. A baby who hasn't been deemed by nature and 'The Unseen' as fit to arrive on Sori Island need not apply for membership to the human species here. Twins, especially, are not welcome and women who call them forth are looked upon with suspicion and fear.

Body Image

The newborn is considered and treated as though it were part of the mother's body for several years; it is bound to her with a cloth, placed ventrally at feeding time, dorsally when the mother is working. It is part of her breasts as it suckles. The mother's body-person is part of *her* lineage. Body-person-lineage-ecosystem are interlocked in a hierarchy of systems and sub-systems. There is no perturbation in any of these that does not reverberate throughout the entirety.

Necks forget, buttocks fear, bellies get angry, eyes go around in metastability of consciousness.[11] These are at least the linguistic conventions of expressing emotions. Whatever a psycholinguist might choose to make of this, one can only infer from observed behaviour that such expressions are metaphorical, which is not to say 'therefore meaningless'. Bodies derive energy from the environment, both material and social, and put energy back into it. In terms of energy and process, danger in the environment lies in trees and stones, specifically those that house evil spirits. From other persons one can expect envy, ritual cursing, sorcery, both local and distant. Ego boundaries do not include exuviae; fecal matter on land is contemptible and belongs properly in the sea. One bathes in the sea, because fresh-water bathing is bad for the body. Blood on the ground is a contaminant and one can become ill unto death (with cerebral malaria, for instance) for having hovered over a place where blood has been spilled.

As long as they did not speak the same language or a *closely* related language, others could be eaten as a meat side-dish for *sak-sak*. 'One-talk' (same language) corpses were sent in trade for credit to groups who could eat them. The Germans, English and Australians put a stop to this, but it is still not seen as wrong to eat parts of an enemy corpse.

When a person died he was dressed up in finery, as though ready for action, and laid on a bed. As the skin swelled the points of rupture would be covered with red paint. ('It really stunk and we had to eat our meals with this stink,' recalled Salai.) All the father's sisters, actual and classificatory, had to wash the corpse daily during decomposition; the bones were then hung to dry, covered with incised dog's teeth. The skull was put into a bowl and the mother's brother's people gave a big feast. 'Cries' celebrating the virtues and achievements of the deceased were composed by the women as they wept copiously as mourners. A man might mourn the death of a beloved wife so grievously that his ritual freedom was achieved by murder, to avenge his loss and to get even with the world. The last one recalled for me was in the 'time belong

English' (after World War I). Ndrakali, a Mokerang Matankor in need of such therapy, talked to his cross-cousin and they decided to *'katim wanfela mast'* ('cut down a mast'), a euphemism for 'cutting down a master'. And they murdered an Englishman who thought they had come to sign a plantation-worker contract.

Discourse concerning the body and body-image is not possible without consideration of shame, anger or guilt related to illness. In fact, all three may surround illness in dense juxtaposition. Potihin, chief of Mokerang, warned me that he had talked to girls who took care of my baby about their irresponsibility. One of them walked the baby to sleep each evening on a road that passed a young man's house. Potihin feels it is a 'road no good'. (I recall that the *House Lotu*, Catholic church, is on this road; Potihin is not a Christian.) Ghosts hover over the treetops on this *tjinal* (evil spirit) infested road. *Tjinal* are specific people, long dead, who have given illness to the Mokerang. Also, my white baby is out too early in the morning before the sun is strong enough; he will get sick from both of these exposures. But they (proud Pwepwe from Sori and that free-wheeling Masian of the arrogant Pere) scoffed at him.

Why do village babies get sick? There are many reasons. Potihin's grandchild had diarrhoea because his daughter Hikwol made her husband ashamed and her husband's sister angry. Hikwol had said to them at a party: 'By what road [genealogy] do you sit at this table?' Both of them wept with shame. Potihin continued, 'We talked and talked among ourselves and with the spirits of the dead. "Hikwol, the wrong is yours, you will pay your husband's family two pounds Australian." The baby was alright then.'

Thus, wrongdoings must be confessed, as among the Pere.[12] Anger gets bottled up and 'buggers up the thinkthink' and to thus impair others is a truly wicked offence.

A person can be shamed to illness in several ways. A woman, for example, was seen by her husband's brother as she was on a tree-top and her genitals were exposed to his glance. In another instance, a man was not paid by his wife's temporary consort for a sexual encounter. Both were undisputed reasons for shame suicide.

In the Mokerang, physical defects in an individual are minimized by the group, so that he may overcome his shame; one amputee is called 'shark', after his 'surgeon'. His condition is a source of village jokes and laughter, but he gains status by this much as a favoured comic in America might do by exhibiting a sub-normal IQ. So too with deaf-mutes who become colleagues with all others in the village in inventing a language; two deaf-mutes were considered 'movie-stars' as I filmed this process. They were often put into hilarious competition with small children to demonstrate that they could be surpassed by the latter. The Mokerang thought ill of the Pere who 'sent back' a bride after she became paralysed.

The Sori were ashamed of the repulsiveness of their sores, ashamed of taking up my time and medicines. Often they would not come until sores were purulent and a stick was needed for walking. Men refused to be photographed for somatotyping, saying that the nude body was shameful. Lohai made an unforgettable comment: 'The white people have come to New Guinea to plant coconuts and coffee, to collect trochus shell, to missionize the natives, to teach school, to sell things. It is all white man's "work", they all think it's all got to be good because it's work. Well, we can't stop them on land and sea but we don't have to give them our bodies so that they can "study" our sickness. We can choose to keep our own sickness and even to die from them.'

The women, led by Lohai's wife Salai, fought this stance bitterly, insisting that the whites were right to learn all they could about sickness, that Lohai and the men were stupid; Salai, for her part, wished the men would all get an unknown disease and die! This liberating speech was given by Salai at a public gathering.

Questions about homosexuality met with stunned incredulity in both villages. They then used me as an informant on such cultural perversity. Did we have such *longlong* (crazy) men because we had too many people and therefore the rules of avoidance, exchange and respect were difficult to keep straight? Did such 'men' have female breasts? Were they really 'men true'?

Leprosy was taken up by the native preachers as the mark of sinfulness in a person – that he drank beer, danced on the church lawn, did not go to church. 'You will have time to think about God on Analawa [the leprosarium island],' they threatened their flock.

Of Dreaming and the Unseen

Admiralties' demography includes the ghosts of the department.

During my stay, Pere village was on the verge of moving its houses again because too many babies were dying of gastro-intestinal problems; the land was heavy with ghosts wreaking revenge for their non-being on the newly born. Evil spirits in the tree-tops in Mokerang village could be seen from a canoe distant from shore. Sometimes spirits stopped at a certain crossroad, lured from their trees by a fisherman's night lanterns or the smell of fish caught by a Bushman. There were many right after World War II because of dead Japanese on the shores.

The only proper way to communicate with a ghost is to contact an old woman medium through whom the ghost will diagnose the illness and prescribe the cure by a binary information system of low whistles, as in the *tilitili* of the Pere.[13] Then there are 'filthy ways' of the Bush folk. The *ngam* is a bush spirit who can be used by one who has been given power while sleeping under a tree or near a stone. *Ngam* are invoked by throwing one dog tooth for each person you want dead into a wooden bowl. The red betel nut was also thrown into a bowl to cause a chief to 'bugger up' and his place to become 'rubbish' (poor). Such *ngam* sorcery can be repelled with the equivalent of the American Indian medicine bundle: lime, leaves and purpur (the grass from which skirts are made). *Ngam* also fear the croton leaf. Since *ngam* live in inland places, it is the *tamberan* (bush shaman) who can use them most readily. A Matankor will be struck by a Bush person who points his lime stick at him with the result that he will get sores on the mouth, neck, cheeks, lose much weight and die. It is always best to travel by daylight, for night lights attract these pests, who also cause baldness.

For *mborokum* sorcery, the agent is food. You are invited to eat, the left-overs of your dish are thrown on your roof ('It will sound like sand falling'). If you hear it you can build up resistance to diseases by beating on your house posts. If you fail, you will not be able to work in your garden or to finish your canoe. At every big feast there is someone among the invited guests who comes with the magic to ruin things.

A person still depicts his dream by going out in the morning and sketching his dream in the sand. There is no other form of communication about the dream, and no speaking; those who watch are silent. But if a man has a dream of a canoe going down there will be no canoes going out all that day. Is non-verbalization a recognition of the non-linear quality of dreams as regards time and space? A dream begets status for the dreamer. An individual's dream indicates his foreknowledge on important issues about the future, as in the cargo cult phenomenon.[14]

Hygiene, Health Care and Preventive Medicine

During menstruation a girl has to eat from her own utensil and dishes. If someone else eats from her dishes her 'flesh will not come up right'. This must be strictly observed before her initiation feast, at which time the women of the girl's totem call upon the totem to protect her. The girl's arms and legs will become paralysed, or she might be sterile, if this precaution is not taken. After menstruation the young girl used to be tattooed; now it is optional. Held down by the women, she was cut with obsidian; she screamed with pain as blood dripped all around her. Burnt grease and ashes were rubbed into the skin; the higher her family's rank, the more markings it was assumed she would bear.

A small child might have his forehead tattooed to get rid of fever and head pains. His face will be covered with black paint if he must be brought near a cemetery so that he will go unrecognized by the malevolent dead. To protect the child's health the parents must not only observe taboos, they must also not steal, become angry, cause anger in others. If the child does not respond to such precautions and therapies, it simply means that he would not have turned out well had he lived.

Epidemics are explained by wind or smoke theories of illness. Wind illnesses leave no one untouched. It does not matter how careful one is, the first time around it hits the children and the second time, the adults. Smoke illnesses are random, coming up from a spot on the ground and affecting only certain individuals. Any illness can fall into several epidemiological categories at once: wind, sorcery, broken taboos, and infections of the white man.

To rest in the daytime when one is ill is pure folly, since it allows the illness to really get a grip on you. You have to walk about, make the blood run and keep ahead of the sickness. ('Have you not noticed, Misis, that when people are really sick they are lying down?') Heads are shaved for relief of headache. Medicines must be just right; not so strong as to remove all your strength, but strong enough to remove enough of your strength to make your headache disappear.

The full moon is dreaded by epileptics and their families. If seizures occur when there is no full moon, such is not noticed, but when the moon is out, causality is instanced. Epileptics had been left, as infants, under a bad tree by a careless sitter.

The Journey

A long illness constitutes a journey of self-discovery for the sick person and allows for the communication of formerly unspeakable subjects and decisions. Matawai of Pere had been ill for nineteen years. He travelled far and wide to find a cure for what he now thinks was tuberculosis, trying all the magic cures of the Manus, the Matankor, the Usiai to no avail. He even went to Tabaul, New Britain. He finally cured himself with a drink he concocted of ground bark of the *yar* tree, ocean water and lime. Two years after he took this drink he stayed in his house, did not go to church, and then he got well. His journey-cure was a saga of self-discovery and medical education. He will now be consulted as a healer.

On the north coast a man becomes a healer by sitting under a tree or near a stone and receiving a visitation by a spirit, who gives him the secrets of healing while they take an imaginary journey together. There are bush spirits in certain trees, particularly old ironwood trees (callophylum).

A Social Definition of Insanity

Hitawari slept in the *House Lotu* (church) usually weeping and calling out to St Mary and the Pope. She had gone to the Catholic school in Rabaul, had come back to Mokerang and married in the church, but her husband was not her choice. She came to my house one night in tears to tell me that her husband and his lover Suzy were plotting to take her three children from her by saying that she was crazy. Suzy and Hitawari's husband, Charles, had a child and looked forward to their marriage, pending the solution of the Hitawari problem. Hitawari was also in trouble with her brother Lokowa because she had said to his daughter: 'You will not finish school since I did not. You will become insane as I have.' This is the *ei* curse. The father's sister causes illness and misfortune through the ritual curse that she has the right to employ (*tendri-teniteni* among the Pere, *giriye* among the Sori, and *ei* in Moker-ang). The sister marries out, losing her rights to property, but re-taining a spiritual hold on her brother and his offspring.

I gave Hitawari a tranquillizer and suggested that she retract the curse in the traditional way, by passing the croton leaf over the parents as they slept. She had offered to retract the curse by shaking hands, the way of the church, but not through the 'fashion belong all *kanaka*'. This was not acceptable to her brother. I found myself sharing her frustrations, accepting her paranoid reality and determined to help her. I asked Potihin if she was crazy. 'Of course not. If she were really crazy she would run around the village naked.' Villagers would instance her insanity by noting that she entered my house to disturb me during my meals, brought flowers and put them on my table, swept around my house, cleaned up the beach (she had learned these tasks at the church school), replied to barking dogs, and spoke of subjects not fit for discourse. She projected her confusion outside of her by waking people up at night saying, 'I want to talk about my right to keep my babies.' The village was not unanimous in its appraisal of her mental status. I myself wavered one night as I watched her bite off Suzy's finger in a vicious fight. But she had been bitten too and came to my steps to bleed and weep. Villagers told me not to feel compassion, for it was better that the 'blood should flow on both sides'. Hita-wari was referred by the doctor. I led Hitawari to a doctor who referred her to a psychiatrist; he diagnosed her as 'schizophrenic' and shipped her to a hospital in Rabaul. Charles and Suzy were free to unite.

I do not know even now whether Hitawari was really 'crazy'. The villagers didn't either. Assessments of her mental status varied with intensity of degree of kinship, and the quantity and quality of gain from her freedom or eventual confinement. Even if clinic-ally insane, she posed a problem in communication in the broadest sense.[15]

In Conclusion

After many years of anthropological field work, I have found it useful to develop a home-invention truth-table of possibilities:

a) I perceive what is going on;
b) I perceive what is not going on;
c) I do not perceive what is going on;
d) I do not perceive what is not going on.

For example, Germans in Sori recorded in intricate and voluminous detail Matankor craftsmanship with obsidian, dogs' teeth, shell and wood; they did not note nor record that the Sori found *them* (the Germans) grossly lacking in delicacy, sensitivity and virtue.

In varied field work situations there always appeared to me to be a context which revealed discrepancies between 'Western' and 'native' categories of illness events and the consequences of conflicting expectations. Notably, the native regards such events as socio-moral and in a class of events of well-being, rather than secular-somatic.[16] However described or categorized, disturbances of the body and life cycle can be considered a ground for universal communication. Communication about health and illness involves not only semantic systems but interactions among them which enter into symptom/syndrome reportage of patient/healer, into causal systems, into notions of perturbation and homeostasis regained. Proprioception is not isolated from other configurations of knowledge. Whether we need to invent new categorical grids for other cultures is and should remain problematic. (Was it not 'totemic' of a French wine-bottler in Bordeaux to identify himself to me as, *'Moi, je suis Barsac, mon beau-père il est Beaujolais'* ?).

Mills' canons of agreement and disagreement do not encumber our Matankor who has his own repertory of facts and determines which are more important than others. The time/space/self modality in which he functions does not require less intellectualization. In this modality, contiguity in time or contiguity in space makes for high probability of causality. The new causal explanation is added to but does not replace the previous one. ('The Australian doctor has come to help our sick babies, but we will make his job possible if we respect taboos and don't get angry.')

As we encounter these people we urge them to worry about the future, not noticing that their present is a celebration of a rich traditional past. *We* raise the question: Is this (mythic) event *in* history? Ahistorical events are real 'archetypes' through which the actual is mediated and structured; indeed such an 'archetype' is a generator (but this is my process-analysis in translation, not theirs). Events as well as things are 'real'; energy gained and lost is 'real'; fantasy as well as praxis is 'real'. For this reason, 'frequency observation' hypotheses (e.g. 'when they count up our medical success stories they will abandon their poor curing ways') fall wide of the mark.[17] Keeping a very sick, non-productive person alive for just a few more weeks, months or years is not their idea of quality medical care. They, if not we, are aware that in their context individual survival *depends* on group survival, which cannot afford to support the heroics of research and clinical trials.

Before we can know the proper levels of discourse for illness, we need to understand imagery and perception, cognitive and emotional structure, how they interlace, and the selectivity and stylizing effects of knowledge configurations which are generated; not only *theirs* but *ours*. Our observations have lacked involvement of intellectual reciprocity. If a Sori uses a reference system for purposes of description he does not imply, as we often infer, that the subject described has acquired the attributes of that reference system.

Information is grounded in the episteme and is purposeful. As soon as I had grasped the configurational aspects of an event and was able to make queries in the proper context and time, so that it had relevance to what was paramount in their thinking, a flood of information ensued. The informant, too, has to grapple with the metaphors and allegories of the investigating culture. He must learn that you also use a reference system which does not reify attributes for purposes of description.

What concerns us here is the 'psychosomatic unit' and illness. The Etruscan notion of *persona* brought about the Roman invention of the legal, moral, economic and political individual. In severing the person from society (and continuing in the severing mode as we learned not only subject but learning style), Europeans severed the mind from the body. This occasioned centuries of vested interests and endless debate on the nature of this duality. Its nature, of course, is a 'mentifact' of conceptually divorcing a thing from its attributes and thereby creating a philosophical problem. But created it was, assuming a dimension of reality which 'caused' minds to mysteriously inhabit bodies and to continue their existence after the bodies disintegrated. Bodies, we still assume, operate in causality systems, without input from minds, a major premise of most 'scientific' medical practice and research today. The science of the investigating culture has a mythopeosis of its own. We are proud that our scientific methods are self-corrective processes, yet we demand unquestioning faith of everyone alive and unborn at any point of the trajectory towards total knowledge, whether those points are at the peak of elegant correctness, or in the valleys of gross and costly error.

Daily opportunities for system-tampering, costly in terms of well-being of the species, are often cast in cultural terms. 'Culture' as an explanatory device is necessary but not sufficient. Before Zen, it is said, a mountain is just a mountain. On the Zen path, it is a vehicle for many allegories of the problem-self; but after Zen, a mountain is just a mountain. It is you (the seeker) who are changed. Mastery of the science of culture must change the investigator, so that he may return to know. The alternative, as Francis Huxley pointed out, is to continue having our interpretations loom larger than the facts they explain.[18] The investigating cultures must learn to go beyond their own concepts, which are their cultural products, to know themselves as others know them. Illusory as all views may be, we can only then begin a science of systems of illusions, and determine which of our epistemes constitute a culmination of fiction-science and which can lead us to an understanding of the human condition.

NOTES AND REFERENCES

1   The New Guinea-Admiralty Islands study 1963-67 was sponsored by the American Museum of Natural History and financed by the National Institutes of Mental Health (USA). Researchers: Theodore Schwartz, Margaret Mead, Lola Romanucci-Ross. Margaret Mead had worked in Pere Village in 1928 with Reo Fortune and again in 1953 with Theodore Schwartz. The 1963-67 study, however, extended to the whole of the Admiralty Islands Archipelago.

2 L. Romanucci-Ross, 'Conflits fonciers à Mokerang, village Matankor des Iles de l'Amirante', *L'Homme*, Revue Francaise d'Antropologie, 1966, pp. 32-52.

3 Cf. K. Pike, *Language in Relation to a Unified Theory of the Structure of Human Behaviour*, The Hague, Mouton, 1967; R. d'Andrade, 'Cultural constructions of reality', in L. Nader and T. Maretzki (eds.), *Cultural Illness and Health*, Washington, D.C., American Anthropological Association, 1973, pp. 115-27.

4 H. Fabrega, 'Medical anthropology', in B. Siegal and A. Beals (eds.), *The Biennial Review of Anthropology*, California, Stanford University Press, 1973.

5 L. Romanucci-Ross, *Violence, Conflict and Morality in a Mexican Village*, Palo Alto, Mayfield Publishing Co., 1973.

6 Idem, 'The hierarchy of resort in curative practices: the Admiralty Islands, Melanesia', *Journal of Health and Social Behaviour*, Vol. 10, No. 3, September 1969, pp. 201-9.

7 *Hospital Practice*, July 1976, pp. 89-101.

8 D. Brown, *Bury My Heart at Wounded Knee: An Indian History of the American West*, New York, Bantam Books, 1970.

9 L. Romanucci-Ross, 'The Italian identity and its transformations', in R. DeVos and L. Romanucci-Ross (eds.), *Cultural Continuites and Change*, Palo Alto, Mayfield Publishing Co., 1975, p. 221.

10 C. Lévi-Strauss, *Le Totemisme Adjourd'hui*, Paris, Presses Universitaires de France, 1962.

11 T. Schwartz and L. Romanucci-Ross, 'Drinking and inebriate behaviour in the Admiralty Islands, Melanesia', *Ethos*, Vol. 2, No. 3, Fall 1974, pp. 213-31.

12 R. Fortune, *Manus Religion*, Philadelphia, American Philosophical Society, 1935.

13 Ibid.

14 T. Schwartz, 'The Paliau Movement in the Admiralty Islands, 1946-1954', New York, Anthropological Papers of the American Museum of Natural History, Vol. 49, part 2, 1962.

15 See G. Bateson, *Naven*, Cambridge, Cambridge University Press, 1936; T. Szasz, *The Myth of Mental Illness: Foundations of a Theory of Personal Conduct*, New York, Harper and Row, 1961.

16 L. Romanucci-Ross, 'The hierarchy of resort . . .', op. cit.

17 C. Erasmus, *Man Takes Control: Cultural Development and American Aid*, New York, Bobbs-Merrill, 1961.

18 F. Huxley, *The Invisibles*, London, Rupert Hart-Davis, 1966.

R. G. Willis

7

Magic and 'Medicine' in Ufipa

First of all, there is no term in Fipa corresponding to our words
'magic' and 'medicine'. The Fipa word *ing'aanga* means a body of
knowledge, handed on to a practitioner (*sing'aanga*) by a similarly
qualified teacher. This knowledge concerns operations some of
which, because Western science cannot recognize in them any
directly causative connection, would be labelled 'magical', while
others might, though sometimes with difficulty, be called 'medical'.
Fipa theory and practice do not distinguish between forms of
'knowledge' (*ing'aanga*) which are, by Western-scientific criteria,
'magical' in their effects, and those which are 'medical'. We shall
see that this is logically impossible for Fipa, since the operations
predicated by 'knowledge' have a uniform structure. In other
words, the 'problem' raised by the character of Fipa 'knowledge'
is a problem that inheres in the form of *our* thought, not of theirs.
But since this chapter is not about Western-scientific thought, but
about the thought and practice of the Fipa, it will attempt to elicit
the meaning of their behaviour in the spheres of 'magic' and
'medicine' by a consideration of relevant Fipa evidence in the context of the englobing structure of Fipa cosmological assumptions.

Ing'aanga then, denotes a body of knowledge. This knowledge
can be embodied in worked, material substances. A unit of such
worked substances, intended to achieve a specific object (either
'magical' or 'medical'), is called *ileembo* (pl. *amaleembo*). This is
another untranslatable term, the meaning of which this chapter
seeks to elicit by a combination of structural analysis and context-
ual exegesis.[1]

139

The Fipa are cultivators living by a mixed subsistence and cash economy. They number nearly 100,000 and the majority of them live on a high plateau in south-west Tanzania near the south end of Lake Tanganyika. Their language belongs to the 'Bantu' linguistic category.[2]

The essential features of the Fipa world-view are contained in a 'key' myth. According to this myth, the first man in the world, called Ntaatakwa ('the Unnamed One'), fell from the sky at the beginning of time at a place called Milansi ('the Eternal Village'). Ntaatakwa founded the senior chiefly line in Ufipa. Later Milansi was visited by three strange women, the eldest of whom managed formally to take possession of the country by sitting on the royal stool of Milansi. Her descendants, called Twa, formed the junior chiefly line in Ufipa. The myth says that the conflict between Milansi and the Twa was resolved by an agreement whereby Ntaatakwa and his line remained the acknowledged source of all authority in Ufipa, although Milansi's political control was restricted to a small enclave round the royal village, which is situated on the slopes of a mountain, itself located in the rough geographical centre of the plateau; the Twa, under the umbrella of Milansi's ritual dominance, assumed political control of the great mass of the country.[3]

This myth, a story which ostensibly accounts for the complementary division of sovereignty in Ufipa between two major royal houses, can be shown to embody the essential structure of the Fipa cosmos.[4] The complementary and opposed attributes associated by Fipa with Milansi on the one hand, and with the Twa on the other, form a pattern homologous with the attributes associated respectively with the paternal and maternal sides of the kindred group (*uluko*) in Fipa theory about descent. Thus both Milansi and the paternal side of the kindred group are identified with the ideas of seniority, overall authority and control, centrality and fixity – but also with relative 'lightness' and weakness. The Twa and the maternal side of the kindred group are identified with juniority, exteriority, mobility – and with relative 'weight' and power.[5] The same pattern is apparent in Fipa conceptualization of the relation between the human community, as typified in the Fipa village (*unnsi*) and the surrounding bush (*icikaandawa*). Here the village community is seen as occupying a central, controlling position, and as drawing upon and transforming for human social purposes the natural energy of the great stretches of bush outside the nucleated village settlement.[6]

Village communities, though they have a strong collective identity, are not of course isolated from other villages. Single men and women and nuclear families readily move from one village to another, generally utilizing cognatic or affinal links to obtain admission.[7] Historically, the chiefs of Ufipa are said to have welcomed outsiders into the country, and positive attitudes to strangers are inculcated into Fipa children as part of their traditional education.[8]

The Fipa model of the person exhibits a parallel formal structure to that just outlined for Fipa concepts of society as a whole, of the kindred group, and of the village community in relation to the surrounding bush. A central, controlling position is assigned to the intellectual faculty (*amalaango*), associated with the upper body and particularly with the head, *unntwe*. This controlling, organizing faculty is normally in constant interaction with the lower body, *unnsana,* or 'loins', the source of all energy. The heart, *umweeso,* is the seat of the moral sense and normally functions as part of the controlling upper body, or 'head'. In this normal state, in which the person's emotional set towards his social environment is good and positive, the heart is said to be 'white'. But the heart of a person consumed with the negative emotions of anger, envy or hatred is said to be 'black', and in this state the heart functions as part of the intrinsically lawless lower body.[9] The heart thus has a dual function in Fipa cosmological thought: it serves both as a mediator between the intellectual and energetic poles of the human person, and as an indicator of the moral status of that person in relation to others. The heart represents the whole person for Fipa in a sense not unlike that which it has for Western man.[10]

The person (*unntu*) in Fipa theory is a structured entity which analysis shows to be homologous with various supra-personal dimensions of the Fipa cosmos, notably the relations between the ritual and political aspects of sovereignty manifested in the comlementary opposition of the Milansi and Twa royal lines, between the paternal and maternal sides of the kindred group,[11] the relation between the village community and the surrounding bush, and the relation between Fipa society and the external world. Without any further evidence it might be inferred from the existence of this total structural consistency that Fipa perceive the human being as 'keyed into' an inclusive system of which he is himself an integral part. That such is indeed the case is made clear in the explicit theory and practice of Fipa possessors of knowledge, the *asing'-aanga* or 'doctors'.

There are at least 500 practising *asinaanga* in Ufipa.[12] These are men – the profession seems to be exclusively male – who have learnt their craft through several years of apprenticeship to an acknowledged expert.[13] Observation shows the clientele of these doctors to consist both of people seeking treatment and remedies for physical and mental (or what in many cases Western medicine would probably call 'psychosomatic') illness, and other people, apparently in good health, who seek the help of the doctors in obtaining for themselves a variety of desired objects. Fipa have a concept of sickness, denoted by the term *ulwaale* (a sick person is called *unndwaale*), which distinguishes the first category of client from the second. Nevertheless, as already noted, the procedures of diagnosis and treatment have a general formal identity in the case of both categories.

A sick person going to a Fipa doctor may complain either of generalized pain (*ukuceensela*), or of localized pain (*ukuwaya*) in a particular part of the body (*umwiili*). Doctors make a general distinction between maladies which they suppose to be peculiar to the surface of the body and those which they regard as existing inside the body. *A priori*, those in the first category are regarded as relatively minor (they include such incommensurable disorders, from the Western viewpoint, as scabies, syphilis, and tropical ulcers), and may be treated with herbal remedies known to many non-specialists; while those in the second category are regarded as 'serious' and as requiring the specialized skill of the doctor in diagnosis. The distinction between the two categories of sickness is summarized in the aphorism, 'He with skin trouble, let him work; but he who has a swelling, is sick' (*'Uwa upele, akalime; uwa ipute, alwiile'*).[14] The word for 'skin disease', *upele*, is related to *impelo*, a boundary of a territorially-based political unit, such as a chiefdom. This suggests that 'serious' sickness may be seen by Fipa as analogous to an invasion of the body by a hostile force. A well-known Fipa doctor, Mr Matiya Isaamba Msangawale, explained to me that it was the doctor's task in the case of a client's serious illness to identify the intrusive agency which was causing the sickness. In this connection he expressed scorn for Western medical procedures which, he alleged, vainly attempted to cure deep-rooted sickness without first discovering its hidden cause. Moreover, according to Msangawale, there were three 'paths' (*insila*) by which sickness could enter a person. These were the path of the territorial spirits (*imyaao nkaandawa*), the path of the spirits called *imisimu* and *ifiiswa* which represent departed members of a person's kindred group, and the path of sorcery (*uloosi*).

These three 'paths' specified by Msangawale relate to three modes of interpersonal relations in Fipa society: the relation of persons co-resident in a village community; the relation of kindred (some of these relations may coincide with the first category); and the dyadic relations of husband and wife, of lovers, or of partners in some economic or political enterprise. Together these types of interpersonal relation exhaust those normally entered into by the Fipa villager.

Mr Msangawale's statement was made in reply to my enquiry as to how people came to be sick (in the 'serious' sense). From his reply to this and other questions, it became clear that Fipa theory conceives the person as constituting a 'node', joined to other such 'nodes' (persons) by three types of relation which between them constitute the substance of Fipa village society. The person is thus conceived as defined by a dual structure of exchange; as a discrete individual, bounded by the bodily surfaces, within which the dominant and central intellectual faculty organizes and transforms into rational and productive activity the energy resources of the lower body; and as a person existing in relation with other persons, with whom he maintains a continuing communication.[15] In both cases the normal state is one in which the centre – the intellect or 'head' in the bodily structure, the self-acting individual in the second – maintains its central and dominant position within each total system of exchange. In the 'key myth' of Milansi and the strange women the social compact, which is also an exchange of specific powers, between Milansi and the Twa, issues in Milansi retaining its central position of supreme authority over a richer and more complex Fipa society than had existed before the agreement between the two parties.

'Serious' sickness, for Fipa doctors, is what happens when external forces invade a person's body along one or more of the 'paths' linking him to his fellows. The disturbance in the wider exchange system (in which the person is linked to others) manifests itself as a disturbance in the narrow system of exchange (formed by the complementary polarity of 'head' and 'loins'). The task of the doctor is then to introduce into the sick person's body a preparation (*ileembo*; pl. *amaleembo*) that will drive out the intrusive agency and enable the person to re-establish both his internal economy and his normal position of fruitful interaction with his fellows. The purpose of the doctor's intervention is to assist the sick person to regain full control of himself. Fipa theory emphasizes the continuing responsibility of the person for his own health, an attitude crystallized in the aphorism, 'Knowledge (*ing'aanga*) doesn't cure you, it helps you care for yourself' (*Ing'aanga, isuwulwaasya, italuusuungula'*).

The doctor, confronted by a sick person, thus first decides whether his client's condition is such as to predicate the operation of hidden causes rooted in the sick man's interpersonal relations. Such causes tend to be presumed when symptoms affect or are believed to affect the middle and lower trunk, including the heart; when they are reported as 'inside' the body; and when they are persistent.[16] Questioning specifically directed to his client's personal relations, then enables the doctor to identify the posited intrusive agencies (e.g. as territorial or ancestral spirits, or as sorcery).

Having made this identification, the doctor goes out into the bush to collect ingredients which will form the primary constituents of a preparation, *ileembo*. These ingredients are known by the generic term *ifiti fikola* (literally, 'the pieces of worked wood in themselves').[17] Although conventionally called 'wood', they may consist of any animal, vegetable or mineral substance occurring in the bush. They always have symbolic significance: thus two women said to have been suffering from recurrent 'dizziness' were treated by Msangawale with a preparation which included as its primary ingredient a piece of swallow's nest, symbolic of fixity and self-containedness.[18]

After obtaining one or more primary ingredients, the doctor takes from a bag called *intaangala* a number, up to twenty or more, of secondary ingredients. These ingredients, called *ifisiimba*, 'latent things', 'things that enter in', are held to act with catalytic force, massively reinforcing or multiplying the intention symbolized in the primary ingredient(s).[19] Although not acting directly, these ingredients are also symbolic. Mr Msangawale's *intaangala* included the following items:

Hair from the neck-hump of a he-goat (*icikonto ca nkulu*). Represents effective action (because the he-goat's most powerful butting muscles are in its neck).

Musk-rat (*isweenya*). Represents intelligence, as the musk-rat is portrayed in Fipa folk stories as a resourceful animal.

Piece of a net used to trap otters (*icaasi miono*). Symbolizes achievement of a difficult object.

Piece of an elephant's ear (*akantaalaala*). Symbolizes awareness (because an elephant's ears are normally in constant motion), and literally means 'what does not sleep'.

Mound made by a mole (*impulumba ituunko*). Represents purposive constructive activity.

Alum (*iciluunji*). Because of its white colour alum represents the symbolic significance of 'white' in Fipa cosmology as the colour of intellectual and spiritual force.[20]

The doctor takes a minute portion of each ingredient and puts them on a fragment of pottery (*iciinga*), together with comparably small portions of the primary ingredients. The effectiveness of the ingredients lies in symbolic significance, not in quantity. He then places the loaded shard over a small fire, and burns all the ingredients to ashes. Finally, he mixes these ashes together. This completes the preparation of the *ileembo*.

Up to this point the doctor has performed a series of operations each of which has multiplied, in geometrical progression, the symbolic efficacy of the materials he is working on. Fipa refer to this potent quality inhering in the substances prepared by doctors as *amaaka*, 'power'. *Amaaka* is also an intrinsic, non-symbolic quality of human beings and animals, and of spiritual agencies. The series of operations begins with the doctor going into the bush to find the primary ingredients. This act is itself potently symbolic, since it rehearses the cosmological pattern in which, in separate but concordant and co-present dimensions, the Milansi chiefdom, the paternal side of the kindred group, the village community, and the intellectual faculty within the person, exert control over a subordinate region which is the source of powerful energy. The doctor's next operation, his selection of the catalytic secondary ingredients, is held by Fipa to result in greatly increasing the force of the original intention, as symbolized in the primary ingredients. Then, by burning the ingredients, he transforms them from natural to cultural substances, so that the final preparation is again infused with symbolic power generated by the doctor's further re-enactment of the Fipa cosmological paradigm.

The next series of operations performed by the doctor is designed to bring the power inherent in the completed preparation into contact with the client. There are several ways in which this can be done. The preparation may be mixed in water and drunk, used as a lotion or made into a poultice; or it may be rubbed into incisions made in the client's skin by the doctor. The last method is the most common and the one invariably employed in cases of 'serious' sickness involving treatment of intrusive agencies, sometimes in conjunction with other methods.

These incisions, called *innkalo,* are made with a razor. The doctor holds a piece of his client's skin between his left forefinger and thumb and makes a small cut with the razor, just sufficient to draw blood. A succession of these small cuts is made, parallel to each other, so as to form a line. Then the powdered black ash of the *ileembo* is rubbed into the cuts. In a day or two the skin heals, and the *ileembo* remains in the client's body.

Such incisions can be made over the site of a localized abdominal pain; but in addition, and in the case of generalized 'serious' sickness, they are made at certain conventional points on the body surface. Two of the most important of these locations are a point over the diaphragm called *apa kameme* and an opposite point over the spine called *apa ntindi.* Other important points are the centre of the forehead (*apa ceeni*), the temples (*apa insasa*), the back of the neck (*apa ngaalo*); less important points are between the thumb and forefingers of both hands, the backs of both wrists, and between the big toe and first toe of both feet. Of these points, the first two are the only ones which do not correspond with visible points of juncture between bodily contours. Their positioning in front of and behind the heart on the bodily surface suggests a connection with the symbolic function of that organ as the centre of the whole person. The symmetrical positioning of these points also suggests the overall purpose of the doctor's treatment as an attempt to restore order to the two dynamic systems, one localized in the body, the other an invisible network of social relations, which together constitute the person for Fipa.

So far I have described measures taken by Fipa doctors which could broadly be called 'medical' in their intention of correcting physical or mental disorder in their clients.[21] But in addition to diagnosing and treating evident or putative pathological conditions, a large part of the average doctor's practice is concerned with meeting people's requests for treatment that will make them more socially effective. All doctors dispense preparations which supposedly improve male sexual potency (*ucoosi*; literally, 'manhood') and female fertility. There is also a periodic need, for instance on the sudden death of a nursing mother, for lactatory 'medicine' which is administered to a female relation of the mother to induce a flow of milk. There is also a wide variety of problems which clients bring to doctors, seeking their specialist expertise in solving them. Clients of both sexes ask for his help in finding or retaining a desired mate; in bringing about the return of a runaway spouse; in obtaining work or money; in bringing about propitious conditions for some hazardous undertaking, such as a long journey; or in warding off injury from others, such as poisoners, thieves or sorcerers.

The formal procedures of the doctor in all such cases is in principle identical with that used in 'medical' treatment. For instance, a male client approached Mr Msangawale seeking treatment that would enable him to obtain a sweetheart. Having satisfied himself that his client had not existing obligations, Msangawale took him out into the bush and returned with two primary ingredients: an ant which had been caught while gripping a fragment of stone in its jaws, and two branches, one from a tree and another from a bush which had been growing under it so that bush and tree were intermingled. The symbolism here of 'gripping' and 'touching' was obvious. These ingredients were mixed with about twenty secondary ingredients taken from Msangawale's *intaangala* ('medicine' bag) and burnt to ashes. The doctor then made a number of incisions on the backs of both his client's wrists and rubbed in this preparation. He told me that the wrists were treated because a man 'used his hands' in taking hold of a girl.

The generic Fipa term for love 'medicines' used by men is *umwiita* ('caller'), which is also the name of a bird forming one of the secondary ingredients in many doctors' collections. It is said a man can put some of this 'medicine' on his tongue, stand in the doorway of his hut and call a girl, and she will be obliged to go with him. Such 'medicine' may also be taken in the form of a lotion which is used to wash the man's face, supposedly making him irresistible to any woman he desires.

Women also make up a substantial part of the doctor's clientele. Love 'medicines' used by women are called *iyaluciilo,* 'husband-spoiler'. Such 'medicines' are said to be able to bring a woman any man she wants, or to make an existing lover entirely subservient to her will. One particular form of this 'medicine' is placed by a woman above the lintel of the room where she sleeps. A man who passes under this preparation on his way out of the room is supposed to lose his sexual potency until he passes under it again in the reverse direction. Or a woman may introduce a preparation obtained from a doctor into incisions made on the insides of her thighs, so that any man who lies with her longs to return.

We can now see why Fipa theory and practice groups in a single set of concepts and procedures what we would distinguish as 'medical' and 'magical' ideas and practices. The treatment of sickness (*ulwaale*), insofar as it is a matter for serious concern, necessarily involves the notion of the sick person as forming part of a cosmic system defined by a common structural pattern which manifests itself in the bodily economy of every human being. The task of a Fipa doctor in a case of 'serious' sickness is to identify and drive out the intrusive agency which is causing the sickness, and so enable his client to re-establish at once both the internal economy of his body and his external economy as a social being. Fipa symbology places the head, identified with intellect, at the centre of the first, bodily system, and the heart, identified with affect, at the centre of the larger englobing system which is also the domain of the whole person.

Persons seeking to improve their situation within the larger, interpersonal system of exchange tend to go to a doctor. His knowledge and practice enable the client, as he and the doctor see it, powerfully to augment the intention already formed by the client as a self-acting individual. In the first case, that of sickness, the doctor acts to restore the position of his client within a larger system; and in the second, to reinforce it. In both cases the doctor seeks first to discover the situation of his client in relation to the invisible interpersonal links by and through which, according to Fipa theory, he is constituted. Having obtained this information he proceeds, through the repertoire of traditional concepts and procedures available to him, to act on his client's bodily economy in such a way as to achieve the desired result within the larger system of interpersonal exchange in which his client is engaged.

Practical 'Medicine'

Some words should also be said, when considering Fipa 'medicine', about practical measures commonly taken by lay Fipa to alleviate or prevent sickness and disease. These measures belong to traditional lore in the same way as proverbs (*imiluumbe*) and stories (*ifilaayi*) which embody the conventional wisdom of the people are transmitted from the older to the younger in the course of everyday life. For instance, muscular pain is often treated by a form of massage called *ukutoonya,* performed by leaning over the patient, arms extended and nearly vertical, the palms downward, and bearing rhythmically upon the affected parts. This skill is taught by parents to their children, as need arises, and after puberty is practised as occasion requires between friends, spouses and lovers.

Constipation is treated by administration of herbal purgatives (*inyeengo*) and in severe cases by a herbal enema, blown into the patient's rectum through a reed, a process called *ukwiinika.* Ulcers are commonly sprinkled with a preparation made from dried herbs, and eye infection is treated with sap drawn from the leaves of a certain tree.[22]

Certain gynaecological conditions are also treated by some of the more knowledgeable old women in each village community, the *amaloombwe,* who also act as midwives. These conditions include menstrual disorders, which may be treated with a combination of an oral potion and vaginal irrigation (when the 'medicine' is introduced through a reed by the *ukwiinika* method), and some kinds of putative infertility, when the cause is believed to be a vaginal tumour. Such excrescences may be surgically removed by the *amaloombwe,* after softening by the application of herbal remedies.[23]

These and other curative measures are applied in the households of the patients. If they fail, or symptoms arouse particular concern, the sufferer will usually resort to a recognized doctor for expect diagnosis and treatment. It is in this situation that the complex of ideas and attitudes described in this chapter becomes operational and explicit.

NOTES AND REFERENCES

1 The concept denoted by *ileembo* seems to be similar to that usually rendered as 'medicine' in the ethnography of many non-industrial societies. See L. B. Glick, 'Medicine as an ethnographic category: the Gimi of the New Guinea highlands', *Ethnology,* Vol. 6, 1967, pp. 31-56.

2 The field research on which this article is based was carried out in Ufipa (the country of the Fipa) in 1962-64 and 1966. The first visit was financed by an Emslie Horniman Anthropological Scholarship grant and the second by the Wenner-Gren Anthropological Foundation. I wish to express my profound gratitude to both these bodies for their generous support. Earlier drafts of this article were presented to seminars organized by the Department of Social Anthropology, University of Edinburgh in 1974, and by the British Association for the Advancement of Science, in August 1975, at the University of Surrey. I am grateful for critical comments and suggestions made on these two occasions.

3 The plateau measures about 150 miles long and varies in breadth from fifty to thirty miles.

4 I here maintain that demonstration of a high degree of internal coherence, such as Fipa cosmological structure can be shown to have, is itself a sufficient guarantee of the existential status of the posited structure. In this way I sidestep the vexed epistemological question of whether, and to what extent, the structure is 'real' for the people concerned, in this case the Fipa.

5 R. G. Willis, 'The head and the loins: Lévi-Strauss and beyond', *Man,* Vol. 2, No. 4, 1967, pp. 519-34.

6 Idem, *Man and Beast,* London, Hart-Davis, MacGibbon Ltd., 1974, pp. 74-9. Fipa villages are densely concentrated, and normally separated from other villages by distances of from two to five miles. Because of their development of a highly productive system of compost mounding, Fipa are able to maintain spatially stable villages over long periods. The average village population of 250 is also about two-and-a-half times that reported for the frequently shifting villages of the nearby Bemba, who practise a form of slash-and-burn agriculture.

7 The residence rule on marriage is virilocal – i.e. brides go to live with their husbands rather than vice-versa.

8 R. G. Willis, *Man and Beast,* op. cit., pp. 102-3.

9 Idem, 'Pollution and paradigms', *Man,* Vol. 7, No. 3, 1972, p. 371. The prototype of such a person is the sorcerer (*unndoosi*), a possessor of knowledge (*ing'aanga*) who has perverted his craft to he service of evil, antisocial ends.

10 The head, *unntwe,* can also stand for the person (*unntu*) in Fipa thought. But whereas the head in this sense represents the discrete individual, the heart symbolizes the person in the totality of his relations with other persons.

11   These sides are called by Fipa respectively 'head' (*unntwe*) and 'loins' (*unnsana*). See R. G. Willis, 'The head and the loins: Lévi-Strauss and beyond', op. cit.

12   This is a conservative estimate based on my own observations. Most of the 1,000 or so villages of Ufipa have a *sinaanga* either in residence or living within a few miles' distance.

13   There is no corporation or guild of doctors in Ufipa. Nevertheless, their ideas and practice are essentially similar. See also J. M. Robert, *Croyances et Coutumes Magicoreligieuses des Wafipa Païens*, Tabora, Tanganyika, Tanganyika Mission Press, 1949. Most of the material which follows was obtained from one particularly well-known doctor in central Ufipa, Mr Matiya Isaamba Msangawale, who was kind enough to allow me stay as his guest at Makansaka village for several visits of several days at a time, to permit me to observe his consultation with clients, and to explain both his general ideas and the significance of his practice in particular cases.

14   R. G. Willis, 'Pollution and paradigms', *Man,* Vol. 7, No. 2, 1972, p. 374.

15   Idem, *Man and Beast,* op. cit., pp. 89-93, where I have sought to show that the act of speech is the paradigmatic form, for Fipa, of the exchange process between individuals in society.

16   Idem, 'Pollution and paradigms', op. cit., p. 374.

17   The Fipa language distinguishes *ifiti,* 'worked wood', from *imiti,* 'timber', 'trees'.

18   R. G. Willis, 'Pollution and paradigms', op. cit., p. 372.

19   The Fipa division of ingredients used by doctors into two categories appears to form part of a much more widespread system of thought in Bantu Africa. Thus, H. Cory, 'The ingredients of magic medicines', *Africa,* Vol. 19, No. 1, 1949, pp. 13-32, says the Sukuma of north-east Tanzania divide ingredients of 'magic medicines' into two classes: those which represent the client and those which activate the 'medicine'. A. I. Richards, *Land, Labour and Diet in Northern Rhodesia,* London, Oxford University Press, 1939, p. 343, implies that the Bemba of north-eastern Zambia divide 'medicines' into two similar categories.

20   White is the symbolic colour of the sky and hence is associated with the Milansi chiefship, with 'up', seniority, the upper body, etc.

21   For several examples of cases and treatment, see R. G. Willis, 'Pollution and paradigms', op. cit., pp. 372-4.

22   I neglected to record the name of this tree, the leaves of which contain a milky fluid.

23   See J. M. Robert, op. cit., p. 93.

Una Maclean

8

Choices of Treatment Among the Yoruba

Illness has always been part of the human condition and, in every culture, ways have been devised for evading or deflecting its ravages and reducing the anxiety which it inevitably occasions. Any condition which interferes seriously with personal plans and reduces one's capacity to perform the normal activities of daily living affects not merely the individual victim of misfortune but reverberates throughout the entire social network of which he is a part, involving changes in the roles of many others who must partly compensate for his enforced inactivity. For the patient, a serious illness carries with it the underlying fear of death or permanent disability and constitutes a crisis which requires co-operative efforts, both from family members and from the accredited local specialists in physical or spiritual care. There are many ways in which reactions to illness resemble one another in societies which otherwise seem widely dissimilar. For example, regardless of the demonstrable pharmacological efficacy of one form of therapy rather than another, merely to embark upon a treatment regime which is acceptable to all one's relatives and friends supplies the satisfaction which comes from social conformity. Moreover, the confident naming of an illness, or its equivalent, the pronouncement of a diagnosis, will go some way towards reducing the fearful uncertainty which comes from the sense of being assailed by unknown terrors.

It is only comparatively recently that Western medicine has discovered effective remedies and drugs which can cure or at least modify the course of many illnesses. For hundreds of years phys-

icians everywhere relied upon complicated and obnoxious concoctions and elaborate procedures which at best were merely pal-
liative and, at worst, both painful and debilitating. However, long
before the science of bacteriology had developed or the pharmacological discoveries of this century had supplied the medical profession with efficacious weapons against disease, doctors were held
in high esteem. The respect which they were accorded derived in
part from their charismatic authority, their association with the
forces of life and death, and partly from their superior knowledge
of matters mysterious to the ordinary layman. We have now
passed beyond the period when the germ theory of disease seemed
all important and we can take for granted the conquest of many
epidemic infections which imperilled our ancestors. In fact, a
careful consideration of the rise and fall of certain common
infections including, for instance, scarlet fever and tuberculosis,
shows that they were already on the wane before the arrival of
antibiotics. Improvements in the general standard of living, particularly as regards nutrition, sanitation, a pure water supply and
better housing, can all be given more credit for the average state
of health of people in contemporary Western society than improvements in the ministrations of their doctors.

At the present stage, with some notable achievements to its
credit and with continuing public faith in its potentialities, modern
medicine finds itself confronted with a number of problems which
are partly of its own making. We live much longer and suffer, in
consequence, from the degenerative diseases which are a concomitant of ageing. And we have begun to recognize the importance of social and psychological factors both in the occurrence of
disease and in the processes of care and cure. We are aware that
bad interpersonal relations can make us feel ill; we realize that the
death of a loved relative can for a time make our own demise more
likely; we acknowledge that patients' return to health can take
place more rapidly in an atmosphere of sympathy and caring. We
have been late in coming to these realizations about the mutual involvement of mind and body, partly because the initial successes of
modern medicine were built upon a mechanistic model which
either assumed a dichotomy between body and mind or even pro-
ceeded on the assumption that bodily diseases could be managed
virtually without reference to the person experiencing them.

But to many other peoples our distinction between physical and

mental illness and our separation of the individual from his social
nexus are meaningless, and they have not even made a distinction
between sickness and other severe misfortunes.

Before examining some of the beliefs and practices relating to
health and disease among the Yoruba of Nigeria, one further similarity in the common human responses to sickness needs to be
noted. A frequent finding relates to an accepted gradation of
symptoms and signs of malfunctioning, from those which are
familiar, non-threatening and susceptible to simple, well-tried
home remedies on the one hand, to those which require the attentions of various grades of specialists on the other. Just as we are
accustomed to try homely cures for the common cold, or request
a suitable cough mixture from the chemist whilst reserving our
demands upon doctors for what we judge to be more threatening
conditions, so we often discover that there exist a range of remedies
and advisers from amongst whom people in other cultures make
judicious choices.

The Yoruba are a tribe who straddle the accidental territorial
divisions of colonialism, living in Dahomey as well as in adjoining
Nigeria. It has always been their habit to dwell in large settlements.
Although in terms of population size some of these could be called
cities, they still retain many of the occupational features of villages.
Ibadan, where this research into traditional medicine was carried
out, manifests what has been described as 'traditional urbanism',
the bulk of the male population being farmers and artisans. The
Yorubas form over 90 per cent of the Ibadan population and,
although 65 per cent would proclaim they were Moslem whilst the
remainder would profess Christianity, traces of paganism still persist, with its connotations of Orisha worship, faith in divination
and a belief in witchcraft. The advent of serious illness or misfortune is especially liable to encourage a return to the traditional
specialists and remedies which sustained generations of their fore-
fathers.

The city is well provided with modern medical facilities since it
has a large and prestigious teaching hospital, as well as several
smaller hospitals and clinics, and a dozen or so 'Western-trained'
doctors in private practice. At the same time however, there is
available a wide range of alternative treatment sources. When an
investigation was made, in the mid 1960s, into the sickness behaviour of two contrasting groups in the population the extent of

traditional medical practices soon became apparent. On the one hand, there are two broad divisions of native Yoruba healers, the *onishegun* or herbalists and the *babalawo* or priests of the Ifa cult, who specialize in what could roughly be compared to a type of psychotherapy. The distinction between these specialists is not absolute, however, since some *babalawo* recommend the collection and preparation of herbal constituents for their prescriptions whilst certain herbalists also practise divination procedures. It would be true to say that the *babalawo* are somewhat more revered than the *onishegun*. But both kinds of healers have to undergo a long period of apprenticeship, learning the efficacy and appropriate use of large numbers of herbal and other constituents of medicines or, in the case of the *babalawo*, committing to heart a lengthy sequence of verses connected with the worship and manipulation of *Ifa* (fate).

In many small shops and in the markets small printed booklets can be found in which are listed a selection of remedies for every ill mankind is heir to. These often complicated prescriptions provide precise advice on such matters as how to secure the return of a deserting wife; how to seduce a desirable virgin; how to succeed in a forthcoming examination; and how to outwit a rival for employment; as well as mixtures for improving potency; ensuring a desired conception; lightening the pains of labour; and treating an ailing child. The prescriptions represent a fascinating combination of empiricism and sympathetic magic. Certain of the herbs may indeed have a pharmacological action, but others seem to be included by reason of a symbolic affinity to a diseased organ.

During the mid 1960s a series of investigations was carried out, in the city of Ibadan and the surrounding countryside, into attitudes to traditional and Western medicine. In the first place, a study was made of sickness behaviour amongst householders in one ward of Old Ibadan, which was traditional in its architectural style, and among families who had been able to afford to send their children to secondary schools in the town. An additional research project involved interviews with one hundred Ibadan herbalists and *babalawo*. The third study was concerned with contrasting methods of childrearing adopted by mothers in the city and those who lived in the village of Idere, some fifty miles to the north-west. Data obtained in these ways were supplemented by observations in local markets, where medicines of all kinds are familiar commodities upon the trading scene; by interviews with certain enterprising herbalists who had evolved into purveyors of bottled 'medicines'; and by visits to the Hausa barber surgeons, as well as by the study of translations of Yoruba medical 'literature'.

Household Survey

In the first phase of this research programme an adult representative from each household in a ward with a population of just over 6,000 was interviewed in Yoruba by a team of University students. Information regarding the informant, in respect of age, sex, family position, occupation and education was followed by a series of questions about the behaviour of the family in the general event of illness. They were first asked about what action would be taken in regard to certain specific diseases or symptoms, namely, fever, convulsions in children, jaundice and smallpox. Next, those conditions which informants considered to be best treated at home were listed. Conversely, they were required to specify illnesses or injuries partticularly suited to hospital care. Additional questions were concerned with the patronage of any kinds of traditional healers and with the extent of that household's use of hospitals.

Four hundred men, as heads of households, answered the questionnaire, and 106 women, in the absence of the male head. Fifty-eight per cent of the men and 86 per cent of the women were illiterate. The majority of the men were artisans or farmers whilst 90 per cent of the women were traders. There were twelve traditional practitioners in the sample of men.

A total of 71 per cent of households reported the use of traditional remedies, either 'sometimes' or 'always'. Invariably usage was directly related to the age of the informant, the number never using such remedies being highest in the youngest age group. None of the people who had been educated beyond primary school stage said that their families always used traditional medicines, whereas 12 per cent of the illiterate groups used traditional methods of treatment alone. Regardless of age or education, an average of 60 per cent of this population stated that they were still using local medicines on occasions.

However, the usefulness of proprietary medicines was also appreciated, being used by 93 per cent of the local families. The drugs in question were mainly febrifuges, anti-malarials and anal-gesics, with the addition of tonics, liver pills, blood purifiers and embrocations.

The majority of the male informants were responsible for pre-paring medicines for their family's use but only a quarter of the women took part in such duties. Although formerly it used to be obligatory for a woman to obtain her husband's permission before taking a child to hospital, less than half of the informants said that this was necessary nowadays.

Half the families reported consultations with traditional healers. However, the proportion with experience of hospitals was much higher, over 90 per cent. Eleven of those who denied any experi-ence of hospitals belonged to faith-healing cults and five were themselves traditional practitioners.

Regarding the appropriate treatment for specific conditions, the use of an infusion of nicotine for childhood convulsions was com-mon. The two basic ingredients of '*agbo tutu*' ('the cold medicine', i.e. not heated) were urine plus green tobacco leaves, but other materials were sometimes included. The mixture was used as a prophylactic in many households, being administered every morn-ing. Children having fits were given much larger doses which could induce coma.

Fevers of all kinds are exceedingly common in Ibadan and European remedies had a large vogue, but 35 per cent of people still used their own household, herbal treatments. Approximately equal groups of households would use traditional or European treatments for jaundice, a relatively common symptom denoting liver disease.

But it was in relation to smallpox that adherence to tradition was strongest. There had been a major epidemic in Ibadan in 1957, and this disease was rightly dreaded by all. Many refused to use the Yoruba name, Shopanna or Sakpata, of the awesome god of smallpox. It was generally agreed that a special ointment should be used on the patient's body. Appropriate incantations were to accompany its use. A particular soap was recommended, but the patient should not be washed too soon. Although injections are generally popular, some attributed the failure of hospital treat-ment to their use in smallpox; however, a form of local treatment in which dried medicinal powder was rubbed into incisions was acceptable.

Many mentioned the use of palm wine, both as a drink for the patient and as an offering to the smallpox deity. Some advised additional sacrifices of cooked beans and corn. In all, equal percentages advised traditional treatment alone or European treatment alone. During epidemics this ambivalence had caused the health inspectors much trouble, since many families chose to hide cases of the infection in compounds or churches.

A wide variety of symptoms and illnesses were quoted as being particularly susceptible to home care. On the one hand were mild illnesses such as headaches, stomach aches and fevers. Twenty-six people were explicit about the fact that mental illness could not benefit from European medicine. It was said by some that 'hospitals can treat all diseases except smallpox and madness,' thus indicating the belief that Shopanna, the god of smallpox, was responsible for serious mental disturbances as well as physical illness.

Eight people warned of the inadvisability of taking to hospital those whose illness was due to witchcraft. Among the other conditions quoted as being unsuitable for hospital treatment were impotence, barrenness, swollen testicles, gonorrhea and disorders of menstruation – all of them related to the reproductive system whose correct functioning was the centre of universal concern.

In the course of answering, many people expressed the sentiment that, if it was one's fate to die, no treatment would avail. Some informants indicated that hospitals should only be used as a last resort. Others explained that, if the hospital's medicine proved useless, it would be necessary to return home. One Catholic frankly admitted the use of every available kind of therapy, including prayer healing and local medicine.

Some of the older men did deplore the tendency of modern young women to go to hospitals for delivery and to take their small children there subsequently. Not surprisingly, people's personal experience often influenced their views. Whilst some had enjoyed a complete cure, others only recalled the incivility they had suffered at the hands of the hospital employees and they had determined never to submit themselves to such indignities again.

Survey Among Secondary School Children

Ibadan pupils in the two most senior forms of all the city's high schools completed a modified form of the questionnaire which interviewers had administered to the traditional households. These pupils were from the educated élite, 44 per cent of their fathers being civil servants, politicians, pastors, engineers, lawyers and so forth, whilst only 30 per cent were farmers or traders. Their mothers were mostly engaged in trading (61 per cent), however, although 16 per cent had trained as teachers or nurses.

Among this group, nearly 60 per cent reported that traditional medicines were 'sometimes' used in their families, a figure equal to that found in the poor area of town. There was no difference in respect of the reported use of such remedies according to whether the father was literate or illiterate. However, in those households where the mother had received some specialized job training the family was much less likely to employ traditional treatments than if the mother was in an unskilled occupation.

It therefore seemed worthwhile to explore in rather more detail the patronage of existing folk practitioners by female clients and, for this purpose, a further research programme was initiated.

Survey of Yoruba Mothers

Yoruba women have traditionally enjoyed a fair measure of independence and most of them engage enthusiastically in petty trading. As has been noted, responsibility for the practice of medicine at the household level had traditionally been male, but the sale of materials for herbal and magical remedies is in the hands of the market women.

West African societies have, until quite recently, experienced very high rates of infant mortality. At the same time there has been intense concern with the perpetuation of the family. It is felt to be disastrous for someone to die without sons to carry the spirits of the ancestors. At Egungun festivals, masked ancestral figures dance before the living. Women, although they have no such figures to represent them, are preoccupied with their capacity to bear children and barrenness is a profoundly unhappy state. Even after bearing many children a woman may end by losing them all, leaving the continuation of her husband's lineage to rival wives in a polygamous household.

This study compared women in the ward of Ibadan which had

been the site of the previous enquiries with those living in the rural village of Idere, fifty miles away.

In this case, the questions which were posed covered beliefs and practices relative to pregnancy, confinement and infant care. Special reference was made to the use of local medicines in each of these stages and to consultations with traditional practitioners. In addition, views were sought on a number of children's ailments known to worry Yoruba mothers.

This investigation ran concurrently with an enquiry among one hundred Ibadan healers. Here the focus of attention was upon the mode of their apprenticeship and when it began; their membership of any professional associations; their degree of specialism; their knowledge of the treatment of women and children's ailments; their capacity for dealing with 'diseases due to witchcraft'; and finally, their familiarity with the use of certain specific plants which could possibly be toxic.

Ninety-nine Ibadan women and 108 from Idere were interviewed. The use of folk medicines proved to be universal in the village setting (which had only lately acquired a health centre), but such remedies were less popular among younger Ibadan women. The village women could, if they wished, have their confinements at the Health Centre. But, at the time of the enquiry, few did so. Many Ibadan women, on the other hand, chose to patronize the modern University Hospital's maternity services. Fewer Ibadan women admitted to the use of folk medicines in the course of home confinements than did their rural sisters.

When it came to the matter of sources of advice on problems concerning fertility, there was no difference between the two groups; folk medicine was as popular for this purpose in the town as in the country.

Many details were discovered regarding the management of pregnancy and labour, periods fraught with uncertainty and danger. Certain foods, such as the large African variety of snail, were highly recommended components of the diet and they were also advised to eat mice and tortoises. All these small animals are sources of essential protein in a forest area long bereft of its large game.

A pregnant woman ought not to venture out at night, in case the *Abiku*, spirits of dead children, might try to usurp the child in the womb. Tying a knot in her wrapper would tend to discourage the unwelcome attentions of such malevolent spirits.

Work by a roadside was deemed especially dangerous. Even when sitting quietly indoors the pregnant woman was advised to avoid anyone stepping over her outstreched legs for fear of their influencing the unborn child.

Various herbal medicines exist for ensuring conception, for keeping the child from miscarrying, for ensuring a successful labour and the birth of an unblemished child. Some medicines were meant to be taken by mouth or were for external application, but others were more in the nature of magical talismans hung in a room or about the woman's person.

Many women, both within the city and in the rural village, were convinced that it was possible to induce lactation in an older woman who had once borne children by the use of special herbal mixture. Formerly, a foster mother had been essential for any orphaned infant, but the availability of modern tinned and dried milks seems to have rendered these lactational miracles less common of late.

In the mid 1960s, many Yoruba women still believed firmly in *Abiku* children, whose spirits were referred to above. These children were 'born to die' and provided an explanation for a series of infant deaths experienced by one mother. When one child dies, the next one is given extra special care and names which beseech it to stay. 'Sit down and play with me,' 'stay to bury me' are examples of such names. If a child is suspected of being an *Abiku*, it will not be circumcised at the usual early age; the operation will be postponed till marriage, when the hazards of childhood are past. Special feasts are held for the *Abiku* child and he has extra amulets hung around his wrists, ankles and neck. But if, in spite of all precautions, the child dies, the mother must not mourn but indicate by her apathy the futility of a repetition of the cycle of birth and death.

The birth of twins is, by contrast, an occasion for great rejoicing. Formerly, if one twin died, a small Ibeji carving was commissioned and carried around by the survivor. These carvings, highly individualistic in detail and yet all conforming to a set style, are among the most famous products of Nigerian art.

Five Ibadan women and seven from Idere referred to local deities whom they served. The god Ogun is powerful in war and also a potent aid to fertility. One Ogun worshipper remained faithful to him in spite of having lost all her eight children in succession. Yemaga is the beautiful river goddess to whom women appeal in the early morning, they go silently there and back, avoiding any greeting to passers-by if their wish for children is to be fulfilled.

Traditional Healers

One hundred healers were interviewed in Ibadan. As mentioned earlier, traditional healers fall into two main groups, the herbalists and the diviner-priests of Ifa. The herbalists have acquired an extensive knowledge of the medicinal usage of plants and are skilled in the preparation of medicines, ointments, powders, soaps and all kinds of mixtures. The properties of large numbers of herbs are learned by these specialists from an early age when they become apprenticed to an older expert.

Whilst some of the plants in use do have a direct pharmacological action, in other instances their efficacy derives from a perceived resemblance to an aspect of the patient's condition. For instance, a remedy for impotence may include plantains and a herb with a particularly springy flower stem. The collection of plants intended for use as medicines requires that an appropriate incantation be pronounced. What are termed *Oriki*, praise names, make explicit reference to the plant's medicinal functions.

Incantations are required during the preparation of a mixture and also prior to its use. This is because matter is considered to be powerless without the influence of the appropriate spoken word, uttered according to ritual prescription.

The concept of medicine and its influence extends far beyond the limits which Western usage imposes. It includes remedies or prophylactics which can act at a distance, and charms and counter charms are available for all kinds of ills and misadventures. The idea of preventive medicine is widespread, in the sense of magical preparations which can protect an individual from possible dangers.

Much of a herbalist's daily practice consists of the provision of remedies for common ailments and it is only one stage removed from the knowledge of simple remedies found in every household. But herbalists may employ forms of divination when faced with difficult and refactory conditions. Some herbalists, themselves illiterate, have accumulated lengthy notes on their prescriptions transcribed by a younger member of the family who has been to school.

Divination is the special skill of the *babalawo,* priests of Ifa. Their clientele consists of patients whose complaints are deep seated and persistent, and for whom other doctors have proved useless. They are, in effect, psychotherapists seeking the causes of complaints in the state of their patient's relationships with other people. A complicated divination system involves throwing sixteen Kola nuts from hand to hand and recording the result of their chance fall upon a sanded board. Once a pattern of odd and even throws has been drawn the diviner refers in his mind to his knowledge of the 256 sayings in the corpus of sacred verses, and recites the appropriate section to his client. The message is open to the interpretation of the patient, who will apply its wisdom to his own case.

Among the hundred healers visited in Ibadan, thirty-seven regarded themselves as herbalists; there were sixty diviners, one faith healer, and two who would admit to no label. Only two out of the hundred were women. It was notable that they were, on the whole, an elderly group, nearly 70 per cent of them being over the age of forty-five. It might appear as though young recruits were scarce but, on the other hand, few would claim to have completed their apprenticeship until ten years had passed and some said they had studied for over fifteen years. In twenty-seven cases, the healing art was a family specialty and, though there were few women in this sample, twenty said that women among their relatives were noted healers.

Ninety-five of the group declared that they were in the habit of prescribing for women in labour but only five restricted their practice to women's ailments. When asked about the use of certain specific herbal remedies, most were able to quote a variety of plants to be used to ensure conception, to help pregnant women, to relieve menstrual irregularities and to treat children's illnesses. Fifty-eight declared that they were skilled in treating 'diseases due to witchcraft' and most of these specified a particular antidote for this purpose.

The great majority of the Ibadan traditional practitioners who were interviewed belonged to some kind of professional organization such as an association of herbalists. They were struggling to promote the respectability of their ancient craft in the face of modern competition. This effort has met with some success, in that serious investigations of the composition of the herbal constituents of certain medicines are now being undertaken in Nigerian universities.

Yet their knowledge is still essentially disorganized, being a matter of private and oral tradition. Some have committed a few of their prescriptions to print, and a number of medical booklets were analysed to supplement the information obtained from individual practitioners.

In one such modest publication, details of fifty different medicines were given. When sorted into categories, it was found that twenty-one of them related to sexual and reproductive functions or to child care.

Preoccupations with potency and success in love are understandable amongst the largely male readership of such material. Ten remedies dealt specifically with male dilemmas, for instance:

> Medicine to compel a woman to run to your house.
> Medicine for an unfaithful woman.
> Incantation to be used before intercourse with a woman who has just finished menstruating.
> Medicine to stiffen the penis.

There were seven references to pregnancy and fertility, for example:

> Medicine to make your house full (of children).
> Medicine to cleanse the womb of a barren woman.
> Medicine for stomach ache after childbirth.

The detailed constituents of such medicines and the accompanying incantations which were invariably also given, clearly indicated that most of the medicines were not seen to depend for their effect solely upon the pharmacological potency of the herbal materials they contained. They demonstrated the connection which everyone perceived between medicine and religion and the anxiety to deal with the ultimate causes of misfortunes and diseases. The following 'Words of Advice' from one booklet indicate the part played by personal malevolence: 'We have made this book for the use of all Yorubas, for curing themselves and protecting themselves from the wrath and machinations of wicked people;' and 'We should find out what causes any disease, because most of the things we treat are not causes but symptoms.'

The behaviour of the Yoruba in relation to the crises of their own and their families' lives must be viewed in the wider context of sickness behaviour in the culture to which they belong. Habits in relation to illness and other disasters are part of the process of child socialization, being learned from watching the behaviour of their elders and modified to some extent later by adults' personal experience of disease and of different healing agencies. What a Western-trained medical practitioner might term illness, in the sense of precise physical symptomatology, is regarded by the Yoruba as simply one manifestation of misfortune, something interfering with his personal plans and representing a threat to accustomed routines.

Yoruba medicine is concerned with the identification of all manner of disturbances in an individual's pattern of existence and with interpreting, for its supplicants, the frustration of their fragile hopes and expectations as well as the failure of their physical health. Prophylaxis means the manipulation of fate as much as the prevention of specific disease entities, and medicine can just as properly be invoked for success in love as for protection from an epidemic. Since Yoruba medicine in its broadest sense encompasses the sacred, the social and the psychological, it is proper that its most revered practitioners should also be priests.

However, many illnesses are quite minor. For the individual in any culture the outset of an illness presents a problem of definition; he has to make sense of what is happening to him, in terms of his own past experience and that of the members of his social group. Symptoms will be sorted according to their familiarity or their severity and persistence. Whilst familiar aches and pains will first be treated by simple household remedies, conditions which are threatening by virtue of their strangeness or intensity will demand the assistance of an expert. It looks as though ordinary Nigerian patients use a very similar sorting process to that which we encounter among lay people elsewhere. There is available a gradation of treatments from those favoured in a particular family or by its effective head to those obtainable at a chemist or on a market stall, through the specific and sometimes complex magical mixtures of the herbalist, and so up to the advice of the diviner. Anywhere along the way people may decide that it is worthwhile giving modern medicine a trial since, in the large towns at least, this constitutes a real option. But Yorubas, like other people, are empiricists and will soon detect which conditions actually benefit from Western-style treatment.

In conclusion, why should traditional medicine persist in the presence of its powerful rival? The most obvious reason is the mal-distribution of modern medical resources, which are concentrated in the big cities, the only places where a high standard of care is readily available. In spite of the increasing production of medical graduates from the universities the need is nowhere near fulfilled. However, we know that even in Western society, much mild illness never reaches medical attention but receives self-medication at at home. Most of the complaints which are brought to doctors or healers of any persuasion are short and self-limiting. Once recovery does occur, credit is likely to be given to whatever palliation or symptomatic remedy was employed. Then there are chronic conditions, especially affecting middle-aged and elderly people, which fluctuate from time to time, periods of exacerbation of symptoms being succeeded by remissions. In such instances also, any treatment regime is likely to be credited with bringing about what seems to be a cure. Finally, there is the large range of illnesses in which psychological factors play a part, influencing their outset, their manifestations, and their persistence. In such instances the doctor's reassurance will greatly assist a patient who trusts his adviser. There is no doubt that all these broad classes of illness are also encountered in Africa and will similarly appear to benefit from the ministrations of diviner-priests, herbalists or household experts. On the other hand, some of the remedies used in Nigeria have a demonstrable physiological effect and it would be quite incorrect to consider that all prescriptions are placebos or are dependent solely upon the prevailing belief in their magical power. Finally, the African therapist has for long been aware of the tensions and conflicts inherent in family and village life. The most respected *babalawo* include reference to the wider society, both in their diagnosis and in their treatment regimes. Thus a mental patient who has undergone a period of care in a treatment centre will finally undergo a cleansing ceremony in which his 'hospital' garments are cast into a stream and the last remnants of his affliction are washed away. Thereupon he will participate in a family feast which celebrates his return to society.

It is probable that, in view of the functions they still perform, indigenous medical practitioners of one kind or another will con- continue to play a part in the care of the sick in Nigeria. Their role as advisers on life's problems may persist even when many herbal mixtures have been forgotten or replaced by modern drugs. There could even be a recrudescence of interest in traditional remedies, if health policy workers were to take herbalism seriously as has been the case in China. But the time for this is short as the elderly repositories of oral medical tradition die and fail to be replaced by members of a new generation tuned to the allurements of a very different style of life.

Paul Atkinson

9

From Honey to Vinegar: Lévi-Strauss in Vermont

There is a contemporary fashion for 'medical chic'. Running
counter to the developments of medical science and 'orthodox'
practice, 'unorthodox' theories of illness and methods of treatment are currently enjoying popular attention. Of course, various
sorts of unorthodox medicine have been available for as long as
there have been established orthodoxies against which they may be
evaluated: the history of medicine is littered with 'quack' remedies
and regimes. What is particularly topical, however, is the extent
of general and fashionable interest in forms of 'alternative medicine', as opposed to passing interest in particular fads or fancies.

Such contemporary interest was aptly illustrated by an article
in *The Sunday Times* (11.5.75) which explored 'weird ways to
well-being when doctors can't help'. These included means of
keeping healthy (dietetics, saunas, yoga) and methods of healing
(acupuncture, foot zone therapy). The article was amusingly illustrated by a parody of Rembrandt's *The Anatomy Lesson*: the
circle of onlookers was labelled to represent the different systems of
alternative medicine. (It is not clear whether one should see the
unfortunate figure stretched out in their midst as a hapless patient,
or as the personification of orthodox medicine under assault from
the motley collection of exotic practitioners.) The cartoon was a
very apt one. The optimism of scientific medicine is under attack,
as the wonders of the 'therapeutic revolution' give way to doom-
laden prognostications of 'iatrogenesis'.[1]

To a considerable degree the systems of alternative medicine are
part of what Campbell calls the 'cultic milieu' – that underground

of deviant belief-systems and their associated practices'.[2] For the 'seeker' who turns his or her back on the conventional wisdom of 'science', established religion and organized medicine, the cultic milieu offers a wide range of diverse beliefs. In the medical sphere there are the competing claims of acupuncture, foot zone therapy, herbalism, naturopathy, homeopathy, chiropractic, faith healing and Christian Science to name but a few. In the closely related area of 'health and beauty' there are the attractions of dietary regimes based on macrobiotics, whole-foods, health-foods and so on.

Hitherto, however, interest in such heterodox belief systems has remained somewhat peripheral to the concerns of academic medical sociology. The standard textbooks on the subject reveal this quite starkly: 'marginal', 'folk', 'magical', 'unorthodox' medicine are conspicuous by their almost complete absence, or sketchy treatment.[3] The published register of members of the Medical Sociology Group of the British Sociological Association reveals that, in Britain at any rate, research activity in this area is minimal. The growing corpus of medical anthropology does, almost by definition, take account of medical theories and practices other than those endorsed by orthodox Western practitioners.[4] But here the historical distinction between anthropologists' concern with beliefs in 'exotic' societies and sociologists' ethnocentrism tends to be preserved. As Loudon points out, medical anthropology has also tended to adopt a strongly applied approach, with an emphasis on working with medical scientists towards the solution of health-related problems in non-Western societies.[5]

Medical sociology and medical anthropology both, in their own way, tend to be 'medico-centric' in their dominant assumptions and perspectives. The normal emphasis on the work of organized, orthodox medicine means that, implicitly or explicitly, medical sociologists tend to view the world from within the conceptual framework of orthodox 'cosmopolitan medicine'.[6]

Some medical sociologists have attempted to break free from such 'tunnel vision' by adopting the distinction between a 'sociology *in* medicine' and a sociology *of* medicine'.[7] But even the would-be sociologists *of* medicine tend to remain restricted in their scope of study. Whilst they are more prepared to question some of the taken-for-granted features of medical belief and practice, their quizzical gaze remains firmly fixed on 'orthodox' medicine.

The language which is commonly employed shows how the categories implicit in medico-centrism guide the world-view of much medical sociology (of whatever theoretical hue). The very designations of 'fringe' medicine, 'marginal' practitioners and so on carry within them the unspoken assumptions that we can take on trust the boundaries of legitimacy between the 'core' and the 'fringe' or 'margin'. The conceptual frameworks of orthodox medicine and the social bases of their legitimacy remain largely unexamined. If the themes of fringe medicine are considered at all, then they tend to be treated as bizarre or quaint, and are treated with scant respect. The influential work of Wardwell exemplifies my point.[8] As a basis for his discussion of 'orthodox' and 'unorthodox' practitioners, Wardwell constructs a typology of non-orthodox medical people; he labels them 'limited', 'marginal' and 'quasi-' practitioners. On inspection, it appears that this typology is based on an unexamined medical 'respectability'; the categories which Wardwell proposes as a basis for sociological analysis implicitly reproduce *medical* judgements. Similarly, Wardwell, and others like him, lump together a diverse range of practitioners and beliefs without close examination of the basis of their family relationship. In some sense osteopaths, chiropractors, Christian Scientists, spiritualists and so on are concerned with 'health' and 'illness'. Yet all too often the nature of such 'health-related' concerns is left implicit. Hence there remains the danger that sociologists *of* medicine themselves remain, in Wardwell's terms, 'limited' practitioners – subject to the conceptual domination of organized medicine.

The sociology of medicine is not served by the uncritical adoption of the perspectives of 'orthodox' medical practitioners; sociological inquiry should not be confused with medical evaluations. On the contrary, it should be part of our task to examine the nature of such perspectives; to do so we must suspend judgement on them, rather than prematurely build such evaluations into our analyses. I do not wish to imply that *all* previous work in this area has been guilty of medico-centrism. There is, indeed, a growing literature on 'fringe' and 'marginal' medicine which avoids this pitfall.[9] Nevertheless, it remains the case that the study of non-orthodox medical systems in Western societies remains under-developed and poorly conceptualized.

In attempting to further research in this area, and in avoiding the uncritical acceptance of our commonsense beliefs, or the perspectives of orthodox medicine (the former often informed by the latter), we need to do two things. In the first instance, it is necessary to suspend any prior assumption concerning the *rationality* of any given system. That is, we should not rush to judge any given system as 'merely' superstition, 'quackery', error or fraud. Rather, we should examine such a system with a view to discovering its own internal logic – to seeing how it 'fits together' to provide a distinctive view of man, illness, suffering and health. In a similar vein we should look to how the beliefs and practices are legitimated. In other words, how practitioners, propagandists and apologists seek to persuade colleagues, competitors and clients of the merits of their own system.

By the same token, we should not confine such a perspective to the investigation of non-orthodox medicine. We should, in principle, apply the same principles to the investigation of accepted, orthodox medical belief and practice. Just as we should suspend disbelief when it comes to 'fringe' or 'marginal' medicine, so we should suspend belief in orthodoxy.[10] This is a methodological principle, and arises neither from advocacy of 'alternative' medicine, nor from a desire to engage in 'doctor-bashing'.

Vermont Folk Medicine

I wish to exemplify these remarks in the context of one particular system of 'fringe' medicine. I am not in a position to do so on the basis of observation of non-orthodox medicine; rather, I shall consider one particular *text* which celebrates the virtues of one system. In this chapter I shall examine the contents of a book entitled *Folk Medicine*, by D. C. Jarvis,[11] which was first published in 1960. This book, written by a doctor, purports to explain the 'folk medicine' practised by the people of rural Vermont, USA, and commends the system as providing a regime for healthy living for all its readers. I shall ask how this account of 'folk medicine' provides for the legitimacy of the practices it advocates. Secondly, I shall examine some aspects of the internal logic of the medical system *as it is presented in the book*: I am not claiming that it is a faithful account of the Vermonters' actual beliefs and practices, as if it were an ethnography. I am only concerned with treating the description as an account in its own right.

The basic message which comes across in the book is a very simple one: that a regular dietary supplement of honey and apple-cider vinegar will ensure good health and a long life. Separately, these two substances are recommended for a wide range of physical problems. Cider vinegar, for instance, is especially recommended for those who suffer from fatigue, headache, high blood pressure, dizziness, sore throat and obesity. On the other hand, we are told that honey is of peculiar benefit in the following ways: as a soporific; as a laxative; it relieves muscle cramps; it soothes burns; it helps to control bedwetting in children. Other substances are mentioned in the text (castor oil, corn oil and kelp) but honey and vinegar are stressed throughout. The two substances are commercially available under the name Honegar, and paperback editions of *Folk Medicine* carry advertisements for this preparation.

Jarvis is an enthusiastic advocate of honey and vinegar, and he has clearly achieved some success in disseminating his ideas. The book has been reprinted many times since it first appeared. When first published in 1960 it caused something of a furore in the United States. Jarvis was condemned in the pages of several medical journals; Honegar and promotional literature were seized by the Food and Drugs Administration.[12] Nevertheless, both the book and Honegar have continued to sell. As a commercial venture Vermont folk medicine is clearly an attractive proposition for the manufacturers of Honegar; the symbolic nature of this mixture will be considered below.

Jarvis explicitly presents his 'folk medicine' as an alternative to orthodox medicine. Yet he himself is a qualified medical practitioner; paradoxically, readers are implicitly invited to find the warrant for this form of unorthodox medicine in the author's status as an orthodox medical practitioner (the book is subtitled 'a doctor's guide to good health'). Yet Jarvis also draws a contrast between his own training in medicine and the 'folk' system he presents in the book:

My medical college and internship days in Burlington trained me in organized medicine. When I arrived in Barre, to pursue my chosen specialty of eye, ear, nose and throat, I recognized another type of medicine which I had to know and understand if I was to gain the medical confidence and respect of the inhabitants who lived close to the soil on back-road farms. This folk medicine had not been part of my formal training, but it is deeply a part of Vermont living.

Below I shall consider in more detail the significance of stressing the 'indigenous' nature of the folk medicine. In general, what emerges is a pastoral and romantic view of medicine's reintegration into the rural community.

Jarvis also claims an empirical basis for his use of folk treatments:

> My studies led me to considerable re-adjustment of orthodox approaches. For example, it did not immediately make sense to me that a sore throat could be cured in one day by chewing fresh gum of the spruce tree. But I saw that I would be wise to learn the principles of this folk medicine and cultivate a willingness to prescribe its time-honoured remedies where precedent indicated that they could be as, or more, efficacious than the remedies which organized medicine had taught me to use.

The efficacy of such remedies is attested to and 'demonstrated' throughout the text by reference to numerous cases where the Vermont system shows startling relief or reliable prophylaxis.

Throughout the book there is constant reference to the *natural* as a category which is self-evidently good and legitimate, and folk medicine is repeatedly portrayed as 'natural'. This is done in a number of ways. First, Jarvis appeals to *instincts,* and points to children and animals as acting in accordance with their instincts. Man is portrayed as 'a rebel against nature and a deserter from the animal kingdom'. Yet he is an animal still, and he can learn his natural behaviour patterns from the animals about him – from 'cattle, hogs and other domestic livestock'. Children, too, exhibit such natural behaviour, although most of us soon outgrow it.

Children are said instinctively to seek out foodstuffs which are especially needed for body-building – high in carbohydrates, low in proteins and acid in nature. Many such foodstuffs are sour or bitter to the taste, and Jarvis claims that children are naturally fond of such sour things. (The peculiar significance of this 'observation' will be discussed below.) If we were wise enough to follow the children's example, we would consume such foods ourselves, and we would eat them raw, as tender young shoots. Indeed, not all adults do turn their backs on their instinctive preferences: we are informed that such vegetation is eaten by the rural Vermonters who live 'near to the soil', and who benefit from a normal diet of leafy salads containing these varieties of greenery.

At the level of ontogeny, then, we are told that man can lose his natural tendencies to good health, though the process is reversible. The argument is paralleled at the level of phylogeny. Collectively, man is degenerate insofar as he cuts himself off from his 'natural' roots. As a result, Jarvis maintains, urban man degenerates far more quickly than does his counterpart in rural Vermont. Longevity among rural Vermonters is possible because these people ('living close to the soil') base their dietary habits on their observation of barnyard animals: so they rely on such beneficial foodstuffs as fruits, berries, leaves and roots.

One part of the argument can now be outlined. Nature is depicted as essentially benign, furnishing instincts for healthy living. On the other hand, the natural environment is also portrayed as the source of illness and physical disturbance. The Vermont climate is said to place particular strain on the inhabitants' constitution – and especially on the heart. It must be sustained by a regular intake of honey, which provides a ready supply of much-needed blood sugar.

The Vermonters, as we are constantly reminded, 'live close to the soil'. Just as they cultivate the soil, so they cultivate their own bodies:

> These people accept the body tissues as soil in human form. Management of the soil to its best advantage requires understanding of natural laws, and specific care to maintain and rebuild it.

In other words, ill health is environmental in origin – it reflects the way in which Nature works on Man. Good health, on the other hand, is analogous to cultivation – it reflects the way in which Man works on Nature.

In its immediate surface arrangement, the text of *Folk Medicine* can be read as appealing to a common enough pastoral dream. The shadowy Vermonters who are invoked in the book point to a simple, golden age of horticultural and pastoral life. Jarvis' homely stories, drawn from field and farmyard, seem to speak to the reader from a fount of ancient and well-tried wisdom. It is, we are told, so simple and so *natural.*

The link between Man and Nature can be broken or interrupted, however. Untreated, 'interrupted inheritance produces a change of chemical pattern which, in turn, makes adjustment of an individual to its environment difficult – perhaps for all practical purposes, impossible'. Such maladaption can arise when people find themselves living in conditions which are at variance with 'Nature's plan'. Incorrect diet is one of the most important ways in which Man's link with Nature can be ruptured: expectant mothers, for instance, can spoil the health of their unborn child by eating the wrong things. Folk medicine, however, provides a remedy:

> The . . . expectant mother should take the following throughout pregnancy: on rising in the morning, one tea-spoonful of apple-cider vinegar in a glass of water, taken while dressing. At one meal during the day, two teaspoonfuls of honey in a glass of water, taken during the meal. . . .

Folk medicine, Jarvis claims, recognizes and is based on natural laws, and he is at pains to emphasize its 'scientific' aspect. Given its long historical development, with its origins submerged in the depths of time, it is inevitable, Jarvis concedes, that the corpus of medical knowledge should have become contaminated with 'old wives' tales' and 'myths'. He instances the belief that a child's teething is helped if the mother hangs a necklace of 'Job's Tears' (the seeds of a species of grass) round the child's neck. He also refers slightingly to the 'supposedly magical' powers of asafoetida, thought to repel sickness in winter. In other words, contrasts between medicine and magic, between natural science and superstition are employed by Jarvis in just the same way as they are by advocates of orthodox medicine, or medico-centric social scientists. (Precisely what is counted in each category is, of course, variable.)

The vocabulary of orthodox medical science is also invoked to support the use of honey and vinegar in health preservation and curing. Health is said to reside in the balance of acid and alkali in the body. The main thing, apparently, is to keep up a regular intake of acid, ideally available as apple-cider vinegar, which 'utilizing the whole apple, represents a pure form of ideal ele-

ments'. The vinegar is also recommended as a valuable source of
potassium and other trace minerals. The virtues of honey are likewise extolled – for instance, in terms of its mineral and vitamin
content, and the metabolic advantages of honey sugars over other
forms of carbohydrate intake.

So far I have considered the general themes of *Folk Medicine,*
and I have outlined the types of legitimacy claimed for the system.
It is presented as natural; hallowed by age; simple; efficacious;
scientific. At this point I wish to discuss in more detail the internal
logic of the account, and to examine how the various themes fit together to produce a coherent 'message'. It must be remembered
that the conclusion of the text is the efficacy of honey and vinegar –
or of the mixture 'Honegar' – which are celebrated as elixirs of
health and happiness. I shall argue that irrespective of the medicinal properties of these substances, they can be seen to offer a
logical, and a *symbolic* solution to a number of basic puzzles posed
by the belief system itself – puzzles concerning Man and Nature,
health, illness and curing.

Medication and Mediation

The approach which will be taken in developing this further
analysis is derived from the structuralist style of social anthropology. That style of analysis is inspired by the work of Lévi-
Strauss[13] and his British interpreters.[14] The problem of illness and
physical suffering can be seen as posing fundamental problems for
popular thought, or practical, concrete reasoning (*pensée sauvage,*
in Lévi-Strauss' terms). At one level, the problem of pain and suffering raises the question of Man's relationship with the Divine.[15]
At another level, it can also raise the question of Man's relationship with Nature, and his being as a physical entity. Man's position
is potentially ambiguous in this regard: at one and the same time
he can be seen as part of the natural order, but he is also apart from
it. Paradoxes based on these two aspects are revealed throughout
Lévi-Strauss' work as fundamental to numerous systems of
thought, widely dispersed in time and space. Leach summarizes
this recurrent concern in the following terms:

The concept of humanity as distinct from animality does not

readily translate into exotic languages, but it is Lévi-Strauss'
thesis that a distinction of this sort – corresponding to the opposition Culture/Nature – is always latent in men's customary
attitudes and behaviours even when it is not explicitly formulated in words.[16]

The first theme to be developed in relation to *Folk Medicine*,
therefore, is how it poses the problem of Man in relation to Nature.
Man is portrayed as separate from Nature in two senses, as I have
indicated. Individually, man grows up and away from Nature and
her laws. Collectively, through the process of 'civilization', he loses
his knowledge of natural processes, which then must be re-learned.
Yet health, we are told, is dependent on some form of integration
between the two domains. The major problem to be solved in the
Folk Medicine system, then, is how the Man/Nature opposition
can be resolved and the two poles reconciled.

The first approximation to a reconciliation was mentioned in
my earlier remarks. It was noted that disease is environmental in
origin, whilst health is conceptualized through the metaphor of
horticulture or agriculture. Hence, one form of mediation which
recurs in the text centres on the process of *cultivation*. The natural
component of Man is balanced by the cultural domination of
Nature.

Secondly, we must remember the special place of domestic
animals, which comprise one of the recurrent sources of illustration
and 'evidence' in *Folk Medicine*. Just as cultivation provides an
intermediate ground where Man and Nature meet, so *domestication* stands for another area where the two come together in productive harmony. By means of intermediate categories, Man may
find his path back towards the Natural. Hence, Jarvis places great
stress on the observation of animal behaviour, and awareness of
their diet and habits. Man must 'go to school' with them, he
argues.

Now, while domestication and cultivation provide a conceptual
framework for modern man's rediscovery of health and fitness,
they do not directly furnish a remedy for the ills of urban man.
Further elements in the 'message' must be incorporated before the
precise significance of honey and vinegar can be tied to the conceptual scheme.

As pointed out already, just as man has deviated from his

natural being, so individual men grow away from their instinctive knowledge of natural health. Hence:

Nature : Culture : : Childhood : Adulthood

and it is in relation to this correspondence that the message is encoded in more detail. We are told two rather striking things about children's instinctive preferences when it comes to diet. First, they naturally go for *sour* plants, drinks and foodstuffs. Secondly, they consume such foodstuffs *raw*. Hence what is sour and what is raw become equated with the *natural* categories.

If we take the unstated oppositions to these two components, we generate a series of binary oppositions which are all, in their different ways, expressions of the distinction Man and Nature. This theme, then, is represented through a number of different *codes*. First we identified the code of *agriculture* – of cultivation and domestication. Secondly, we find the *gustatory* code, with its opposition of sweet and sour. Additionally, there is the *culinary* code, where the opposition is stated (or at least implied) in terms of raw and cooked foodstuffs. In other words:

Nature : Culture : : Sour : Sweet : : Raw : Cooked

At this point it becomes possible to discern the symbolic significance of Honey + Vinegar. If health is promoted by virtue of the mediation of the Man/Nature opposition, then we should expect that at the level of diet and medication, a similar resolution of the polarities would be achieved. In the first instance, the resolution is achieved in a simple manner. Honey + Vinegar combines the two gustatory elements (sweet + sour) in a straightforward way – and the preparation 'Honegar' combines them physically in a single mixture.

But is it as simple as this? What of the culinary code? How does Honey + Vinegar fit into this scheme? At this point it is necessary to turn aside to consider the work of Lévi-Strauss. In the analysis of American myths in his *magnum opus, Mythologiques,* Lévi-Strauss pursues a number of recurrent themes concerned with types of food and food preparation in the symbolic representation of man's relationship with the natural order, and the origins of culture.

Lévi-Strauss' exploration of such collective representations shows the use of concrete metaphors for the expression of these fundamental relationships. This is summarized in the following passage:

> . . . natural conditions are not just passively accepted. What is more they do not exist in their own right for they are a function of the techniques and way of life of the people who define and give a meaning by developing them in a particular direction. . . . On the other hand, even when raised to that human level which alone can make them intelligible, man's relations with his natural environment remain objects of thought: man never perceives them passively; having reduced them to concepts, he compounds them in order to arrive at a system which is never determined in advance: the same situation can always be systematised in various ways.[17]

Food and Cooking are two of the concrete systems of activity and classification which are typically available for such manipulation, and Lévi-Strauss examined their use in some detail.[18] It is a human universal that not all foodstuffs are consumed in their natural state (raw). There are cultural definitions as to what should and should not be eaten raw, and, if appropriate, the ways in which food should be prepared and processed. The commonest way of processing food is via the *cultural* transformation which is involved in cooking. An alternative involves the *natural* transformation of 'rotting' (e.g. Stilton cheese). Hence, Lévi-Strauss argues that systems of culinary conventions furnish codes which are available for the expression of Culture/Nature oppositions. The underlying framework is represented in the form of the 'culinary triangle' (see Figure 1).

The vertical axis of Figure 1 refers to the degree of elaboration imposed on the basic foodstuff; the horizontal axis refers to the Nature/Culture dimension. The system is elaborated by taking account of various actual methods of food preparation (roasting, boiling, smoking, etc.), but these niceties need not concern us here.

The basic rationale for the analysis of culinary codes is outlined by Leach:

> In that we are men, we are all a part of Nature; in that we are all human beings, we are all a part of Culture. Our survival as

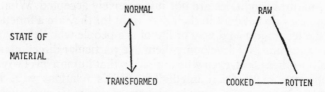

FIGURE 1: 'THE CULINARY TRIANGLE' (from Lévi-Strauss, 1966a)

men depends on our ingestion of food (which is a part of Nature); our survival as human beings depends upon our use of social categories which are derived from cultural classifications imposed on elements of Nature. . . .

Food is an especially appropriate mediator because, when we eat, we establish, in a literal sense, a direct identity between ourselves (Culture) and our food (Nature).[19]

This is the argument which is developed in Volume I of *Mythologiques* (*The Raw and the Cooked*), where Lévi-Strauss detects, beneath the surface detail of American Indian myths, a recurrent concern with the origins of cooking and of meat as a substance for cooking. In the myths concerning the use of fire, there also appear references to tobacco and honey, and the significance of these topics is explored in Volume II of the series (*From Honey to Ashes*).

According to Lévi-Strauss, honey and tobacco enter into the mythic system insofar as they offer a complementary pair of oppositions to the raw and the cooked. They fill out the exploration of the basic culinary metaphor since honey is 'infra-culinary' and tobacco is 'meta-culinary'. By these terms Lévi-Strauss refers to the fact that, strictly speaking, the consumption of neither depends on 'cooking':

For honey is made by non-human beings, who supply it ready

for consumption, whilst the most common method of consuming tobacco places the latter, contrary to honey, not on the hither side of cooking but beyond it. It is not consumed in the raw state, as is honey, nor exposed to fire before consumption, as is the case with meat. It is burnt to ashes, so that the smoke thus released can be inhaled.[20]

Although *Folk Medicine* does not involve reference to tobacco, the diversion is far from irrelevant. Here, of course, honey appears not with tobacco, but with vinegar. However, I would suggest that vinegar can be understood in the context of a culinary system, in the sense indicated earlier. There is a range of methods for preparing foods and drinks which has not, as yet, been specifically mentioned. They are applicable more to drink, and should be placed towards the 'rotten' apex of the culinary triangle. I am referring to the process of 'fermentation' (broadly speaking) in the preparation of beverages (brewing beer, wine-making and so on), including the production of vinegar. These processes clearly involve the human induction or facilitation of natural processes of transformation, which produce reactions closely akin to those of 'putrefaction'.

If we return to the themes of *Folk Medicine,* then, we have seen how the logic of the system is concerned with the Nature/Culture opposition and its resolution. We should therefore expect that the remedy or remedies recommended should in some way mediate between Nature and Culture. Not only should the 'medicine' seek to restore psysiological functioning, it should also ensure a resolution at the level of the semiological system.

Honey and Vinegar do appear to perform such a mediating function. Between Nature and Culture stands Honey – which is 'made' (Culture) by non-human agents (Nature). In a similar position, Vinegar is the mirror-image of Honey – it is made by human agents (Culture) by means of putrefaction (Nature). The relationship between natural and cultural *means* and natural and cultural *agents* is expressed in Figure 2.

Where the congruent elements (Natural/Natural and Cultural/ Cultural) are represented by 'Raw' and 'Cooked' respectively, Honey and Vinegar occupy the ambivalent, 'off-diagonal' cells. Thus, it is apparent that the mixture of Honey and Vinegar offers an ideal medium for the resolution of the opposition between the

MEANS

	NATURAL	CULTURAL
NATURAL	Raw	Honey
CULTURAL	Vinegar	Cooked

AGENTS

FIGURE 2: 'THE CULINARY SQUARE'

realms of the natural and the human. Individually, the two ingredients are alternative formulations of a Nature/Culture confusion or ambiguity. In combination they produce a symbolic 'overkill', but resolve the opposition expressed in the opposition of 'sweet' and 'sour'.

A summary representation of the structure of *Folk Medicine* can therefore be offered in Figure 3.

What has emerged from the foregoing analysis is that there are several codes in which the Nature/Culture antimony and their integration is presented. In terms of the social and physical environment pictured in the text, the imagery is that of a farmyard, with animals, children, and men who 'live near to the soil'. Here man lives by the laws of Nature, thus ensuring his health. The purpose of medication is therefore seen to be the concrete embodiment of such a harmonious resolution. It has become apparent how Honey and Vinegar can do precisely this, by virtue of their ambiguous nature: they are neither 'cooked' nor 'raw', neither 'natural' nor 'cultural'; whilst they are sweet and sour individually, in combination they cancel each other out. Symbolically, therefore, Honey + Vinegar (and 'Honegar') can reunite jaded, urban ('over-cultured') man with the innocent, child-like state of natural grace and health enjoyed in rural Vermont. It offers a concrete short-cut to the pastoral dream of a 'natural' way of life.

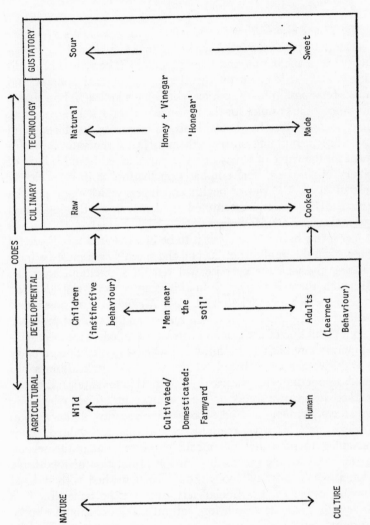

FIGURE 3: SCHEMATIC REPRESENTATION OF THE LOGIC OF *Folk Medicine*

Discussion

So far I have argued that a close textual analysis of *Folk Medicine* reveals that it is constructed according to a number of basic oppositions, their mediation and their resolution. The system of medicine portrayed is based on theories of the natural domain, and man's relationship to it/position in it. I have indicated how Jarvis documents the grounds for the legitimacy of the system advocated. Thus he appeals to its natural basis, its simplicity, its efficacy and its tradition. Building on these themes, Jarvis generates an argument for the value of honey and vinegar, derived from his logic of binary oppositions. The emphasis on 'nature' is in turn closely related to the theories of health and illness which underpin the system. Thus I have attempted to demonstrate the logic and rationality in *Folk Medicine*.

Yet if this brand of analysis is to be of value in a more general sense, then the application beyond the specific case must be indicated – otherwise the exercise will remain a dilettante exercise. Although there is not scope in this chapter to develop detailed analyses which parallel that of *Folk Medicine,* it is possible to indicate some directions in which further analysis might proceed.

A fruitful line of comparison can be extended to consider contemporary emphasis on 'natural' approaches to diet. Such dietary preferences are often based on the supposed 'unhealthiness' of man's tampering with Nature (i.e., cultural intervention); they are marked by greater stress on (and market for) foods which are 'organically grown' or 'whole-foods' – where cultural intervention is weak, and 'natural' methods of growing are valued. It is intriguing to note that the means employed under the second regime tend to rely on 'rotting' in the production of foodstuffs. That is, such 'healthy' foods should be nourished with natural compost rather than 'artificial' fertilizers. At the same time it is noteworthy that the search for 'natural goodness' should also be expressed by a shift along the raw/cooked dimension. For the development of the health-food route to personal physical (and, in some cases, moral) salvation, the emphasis reverts from the *cooked* apex of the culinary triangle to the *raw*. Foods are transformed minimally – washing, shredding, chopping and grinding; cooking is seen not so much as a valued cultural elaboration, but rather as the undesirable destruction of natural goodness. There is therefore a reversion to the consumption of food raw, cooked or transformed minimally. (It is tempting to speculate on the increased consumption of yoghurt in this context: it derives from a 'naturally made' substance – milk – via a natural process – 'putrefaction' – and should be consumed in a natural – 'live' – condition.)

It is thus possible to construct two ideal-typical series of transformations for the production and preparation of foodstuffs (see Figure 4). One extreme is represented by the first system, which corresponds to that taken for granted by most members of contemporary Western societies; it depends on 'cultural' means of production and 'cultural' means for elaboration. The 'health-food' system is the reverse of the former; 'cultural' methods are weak, and naturally induced transformations are preferred.

In their various guises, dietary prescriptions which advocate recourse to 'natural' foodstuffs all provide a concrete solution to the perceived divorce of an over-cultured, and over-civilized urban population from their heritage in rural nature or their primal state of harmony with the natural order. One thing which must be borne in mind is that such arguments should not be confused with what are essentially nutritional, not anthropological, problems. It does not matter, in the last analysis, whether the claims made for honey, vinegar, health foods and so on are 'really true'. What is at stake is that they may be thought to be true. It has been suggested in this chapter that systems such as those described in *Folk Medicine* may be thought to be true insofar as they offer plausible and appealing ways of conceptualizing problems of health and illness, and man's nature as a physical being. The dietary regimes advocated are the physical embodiment of these beliefs, whereby the symbolic solutions are encoded into the world of physical objects. In conclusion, and to paraphrase Lévi-Strauss, substances like honey and vinegar may not only be good to eat, but they are also good to think with.

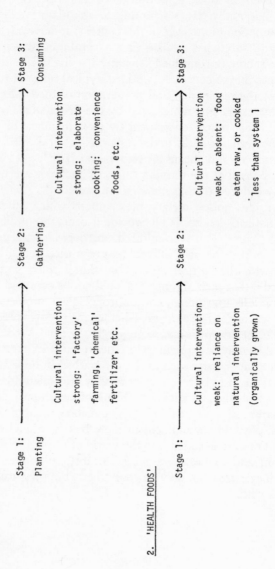

1. "NORMAL" (UNHEALTHY?)

Stage 1: Planting → Stage 2: Gathering → Stage 3: Consuming

Cultural intervention strong: 'factory' farming, 'chemical' fertilizer, etc.

Cultural intervention strong: elaborate cooking; convenience foods, etc.

2. 'HEALTH FOODS'

Stage 1: → Stage 2: → Stage 3:

Cultural intervention weak: reliance on natural intervention (organically grown)

Cultural intervention weak or absent: food eaten raw, or cooked less than system 1

FIGURE 4: TWO SYSTEMS OF FOOD PRODUCTION AND PREPARATION – THE CULTURAL AND THE NATURAL

NOTES AND REFERENCES

1 I. Illich, *Medical Nemesis,* London, Calder and Boyars, 1974.

2 C. Campbell, 'The cult, the cultic milieu and secularization', in M. Hill (ed.), *A Sociological Yearbook of Religion in Britain,* No. 5, London, S.C.M. Press, 1972.

3 See D. Mechanic, *Medical Sociology: A Selective View,* New York, Free Press, 1968; R. Coe, *Sociology of Medicine,* New York, McGraw-Hill, 1970; M. Susser and W. Watson, *Sociology in Medicine,* London, Oxford University Press, 1971; C. Cox and A. Mead, *A Sociology of Medical Practice,* London, Collier-Macmillan, 1975; D. Tuckett, *An Introduction to Medical Sociology,* London, Tavistock, 1976.

4 See J. Loudon, 'Introduction', in J. Loudon (ed.), *Social Anthropology and Medicine,* London, Academic Press, 1976.

5 Ibid.

6 Ibid.

7 R. Strauss, 'The nature and status of medical sociology', *American Sociological Review,* Vol. 22, 1957, pp. 200-204.

8 W. Wardwell, 'Limited, marginal and quasi-practitioners', in H. Freeman, S. Levine and L. Reeder (eds.), *Handbook of Medical Sociology,* Englewood Cliffs, N.J., Prentice Hall, 1972; idem, 'Orthodox and unorthodox practitioners: changing relationships and the future status of chiropractors', in R. Wallis and P. Morley (eds.), *Marginal Medicine,* London, Peter Owen, 1976.

9 See, for example, R. Wallis and P. Morley, op. cit., especially the contributions by Wallis, Allen and Wallis, Nudelman and Lee.

10 J. Roth, 'Ritual and magic in the control of contagion', *American Sociological Review,* Vol. 22, 1957, pp. 310-14.

11 D. Jarvis, *Folk Medicine,* London, Pan, 1961.

12 L. Lasagna, *The Doctor's Dilemmas,* London, Gollancz, 1962.

13 C. Lévi-Strauss, *Structural Anthropology,* New York, Basic Books, 1963; idem, *The Savage Mind,* London, Weidenfeld & Nicolson, 1966; *The Raw and the Cooked,* London, Jonathan Cape, 1970.

14 See M. Douglas, *Purity and Danger,* London, Routledge & Kegan Paul, 1966; idem, *Natural Symbols,* London, Barrie and Rockliff, 1970; E. Leach, 'Anthropological aspects of language: animal categories and verbal abuse', in E. Lenneberg (ed.), *New Directions in the Study of Language,* Cambridge, Mass., M.I.T. Press, 1964; idem, *Claude Lévi-Strauss,* London, Fontana, 1970.

15 G. Obeyesekere, 'Theodicy, sin and salvation in a sociology of Buddhism', in E. Leach (ed.), *Dialectic in Practical Religion,* Cambridge Papers in Social Anthropology, No. 5, Cambridge, Cambridge University Press, 1968.

16   E. Leach, *Claude Lévi-Strauss,* op. cit.

17   C. Lévi-Strauss, *The Savage Mind,* op. cit., p. 94.

18   Idem, 'The culinary trinangle', *New Society,* 22 December, 1966, pp. 937-40; idem, *The Raw and the Cooked,* op. cit.

19   E. Leach, *Claude Lévi-Strauss,* op. cit.

20   Cf. C. Lévi-Strauss, *Mythologiques,* Vol. II, *From Honey to Ashes.*

Notes on Contributors and Editors

PAUL ATKINSON, Ph.D., is Lecturer in Sociology at University College, Cardiff. He is engaged in research into medical education and is an active editor of the British Sociological Association's *Medical Sociology Group Newsletter*.

JOHN M. FOLEY, Ph.D., is on the English faculty at Emery University (Atlanta). He is an 'oral traditionalist' with field work experience in Serbia. During 1976, he was a visiting Fellow at the Milman Parry Collection of Oral Literature at Harvard.

BARBARA K. HALPERN, Ph.D., is a Research Associate in the Department of Anthropology, University of Massachusetts (Amherst). She is primarily interested in sociolinguistics and has carried out research on ways in which collective folk wisdom is retained and transmitted orally. She has extensive field work experience in the Balkans.

DONN HART, Ds.Sc., is Director and Professor at the Center from Southeast Asian Studies at Northern Illinois University. He has published many papers and monographs on medical beliefs, religion, and ethnohistory in South-East Asia. His special interests are peasant societies, folklore, research methods and the Philippines. His latest book is *Compadrinazgo: Ritual Kinship in the Philippines.*

MICHAEL KEARNEY, Ph.D., is Associate Professor of Anthropology at the University of California, Riverside. He has published on Zapotec peoples and for the past seven years has been studying Mestizo spiritualist healers in northern Baja California.

RICHARD LIEBAN, Ph.D., is Professor of Anthropology at the University of Hawaii at Manoa. He has published widely in the area of medical anthropology. He is the author of *Cebuano Sorcery* (1967).

UNA MACLEAN, M.D., Ph.D., is a lecturer in the Department of Community Medicine at Edinburgh University. She spent seven years in Western Nigeria engaged in cancer and sociological research, following that by three years studying social psychiatry in Edinburgh. She is the author of *Magical Medicine* (1971), a book on nursing, and several research papers.

PETER MORLEY, Ph.D., is an Assistant Professor of Medical Sociology in the Department of Community Medicine, Memorial University, Newfoundland. He has carried out research on Canadian Indians, overseas Asian communities, Mexican Curanderismo, and alcoholism in Scotland. He has authored several papers and reports in the area of medical sociology/anthropology and race relations. His present research interests include medical belief systems, social psychiatry, sociology of science, sociology of medical knowledge, and the politics of health-care delivery. He is co-editor with Roy Wallis of *Marginal Medicine,* Peter Owen, 1976.

LOLA ROMANUCCI-ROSS, Ph.D., is Associate Professor of Community Medicine and Director of Muir Interdisciplinary Studies, Department of Community Medicine, University of California, San Diego. She has carried out field work among American Indians, in Mexico where she completed a study of a Mexican village with Erich Fromm and Theodore Schwartz, and participated in the New Guinea-Admiralty Islands expedition with Schwartz and Margaret Mead.

ROY WALLIS, DPhil, is Professor of Sociology at Queen's University, Belfast. He has published several articles on religious sects and social movements. His book, *The Road to Total Freedom: A Sociological Analysis of Scientology* is published by Heinemann Educational Books, London, 1976. He is editor of *Sectarianism: Analyses of Religious and Non-Religious Sects,* Peter Owen, London, and Halstead Press, New York, 1975. He is also co-editor with Peter Morley of *Marginal Medicine,* Peter Owen, 1976.

ROY WILLIS, DPhil, is a Lecturer in the Department of Social Anthropology at the University of Edinburgh. He is the author of several papers and has published *Man and Beast* (1974). He is also completing *There Was a Man: Fipa Stories and Proverbs,* and a monograph *Fipa Society and History.*

Contemporary Community Health Series

Marriage and Mental Handicap: A Study of Subnormality in Marriage
Janet Mattinson

The Psychiatric Halfway House: A Handbook of Theory and Practice
Richard D. Budson

A Psychiatric Record Manual for the Hospital
Dorothy Smith Keller

Racism and Mental Health: Essays
Charles V. Willie, Bernard M. Kramer, and Bertram S. Brown, Editors

Social Skills and Mental Health
Peter Trower, Bridget Bryant, and Michael Argyle

The Sociology of Physical Disability and Rehabilitation
Gary L. Albrecht, Editor

The Style and Practice of a Pediatric Practice
Lee W. Bass and Jerome H. Wolfson